Picture Your
Life After Cancer

The New York Times

Picture Your Life After Cancer

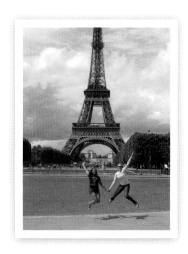

Edited by Karen Barrow

Foreword by Tara Parker-Pope

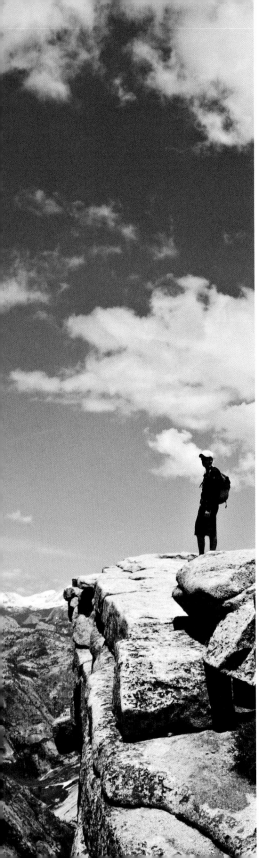

Published by the American Cancer Society
Health Promotions
250 Williams Street NW
Atlanta, Georgia 30303 USA

Copyright ©2012 *The New York Times*

All rights reserved. Without limiting the rights under copyright reserved above, no part of this publication may be reproduced, stored in or introduced into a retrieval system, or transmitted in any form or by any means (electronic, mechanical, photocopying, recording, or otherwise) without the prior written permission of the publisher and *The New York Times*.

Manufactured by RR Donnelley
Manufactured in Willard, OH, in September 2012
Job #28045

Printed in the United States of America
Design and composition by La Shae V. Ortiz

The accounts reproduced in this book are solely those of the people featured and do not represent the opinions of the American Cancer Society. The American Cancer Society does not provide personal medical advice, and the accounts in this book should not be construed as such advice. The American Cancer Society does not endorse any third party goods or services mentioned in this book.

5 4 3 2 1   12 13 14 15 16

Library of Congress Cataloging-in-Publication Data
Picture your life after cancer / the New York Times; edited by Karen Barrow;
foreword by Tara Parker Pope.
    p. cm.
  ISBN 978-1-60443-063-9 (hardcover: alk. paper)—ISBN 1-60443-063-X
(hardcover: alk. paper)
1. Cancer—Patients—Anecdotes. 2. Cancer—Patients—Portraits. I. Barrow, Karen.
II. American Cancer Society. III. New York Times.
  RC265.5.P53 2012
  616.99'4—dc23   2012026394

AMERICAN CANCER SOCIETY
Managing Director, Content: Chuck Westbrook
Director, Cancer Information: Terri Ades, DNP, FNP-BC, AOCN
Director, Book Publishing: Len Boswell
Managing Editor, Book Publishing: Rebecca Teaff, MA
Senior Editor, Book Publishing: Jill Russell
Book Publishing Coordinator: Vanika Jordan, MSPub
Editorial Assistant, Book Publishing: Amy Rovere

For more information about cancer, contact your American Cancer Society at **800-227-2345** or **cancer.org**.

Quantity discounts on bulk purchases of this book are available. For information, please contact the American Cancer Society, Health Promotions Publishing, 250 Williams Street NW, Atlanta, GA 30303-1002, or send an e-mail to **trade.sales@cancer.org**.

Foreword

By TARA PARKER-POPE

Whether you have cancer or love someone who does, a cancer diagnosis is the kind of event that ultimately redefines and reshapes your life. Cancer. The word itself carries so much weight and uncertainty that the moment you hear it, your life is suddenly divided into two distinct parts: what happens before the cancer, and everything that happens after it. This book is about the second part, that is, the days and weeks and months and years after cancer.

An estimated 13.7 million people living in the United States today were told at some point in their lives that they had cancer. Some of them received the news only recently and perhaps are still undergoing the various rounds of doctor visits and treatments that follow a cancer diagnosis. Others are farther along in their cancer journey, having already soldiered through numerous surgeries, chemotherapy sessions, and radiation treatments. The latter group are no longer cancer patients; they are survivors.

And then there are the cancer veterans, those people who are long past the initial diagnosis and treatment but for whom cancer still remains a daily experience. They may be in the late stages of the disease or dealing with a recurrence, taking one day at a time as they learn to live and love and even thrive in the shadow of cancer.

Finally, there are countless others who don't have the disease but love someone who does—a friend, a child, a parent, a husband or wife, partner or coworker. Every person whose life has been touched by cancer has a story to tell.

As a health journalist, I have been awed by the people I have met over the years who have so generously shared their own stories of inspiration and desperation, the highs and lows, the victories and the setbacks that are all part of the cancer experience. They include the late Randy Pausch, the Carnegie Mellon professor diagnosed with pancreatic cancer, made famous by his "last lecture" that inspired millions to dream big, embrace life, and take chances. There is Jan Guthrie of Conway, Arkansas, who has turned nearly three decades of personal experience with ovarian cancer into a clearinghouse of information to help others. There are Nathan and Elisa Bond, a young Brooklyn couple who each received a cancer diagnosis just days apart. Both remain resolute in their determination—not only to support each other through treatment, but to keep imagining a future together, raising their young daughter.

My own cancer experience goes beyond my professional life as a journalist. Cancer has also touched many of my friends, colleagues, and family members. The most profound cancer experience in my life has been the one I shared with my mother. A diagnosis of breast cancer in her early 50s didn't seem to faze her. She opted for a mastectomy, recovered from surgery, and jumped back into her life as if cancer had been nothing but a little bump in the road. But several years later, she found herself on another cancer journey. This time the disease was esophageal adenocarcinoma, a deadly cancer fueled by years of acid reflux and, in her case, one that came with a bleak prognosis.

I formed the most remarkable memories of my mother in the nine months after her last bout with cancer. She approached her disease with a strength and calm that continue to inspire the choices I make in my own life. The grace and dignity my mother showed at the end of her life were her gifts to me. Her unwavering faith in God and family helped her husband, children, and grandchildren all picture new lives for themselves, after her cancer.

In the United States today, men have slightly less than a one in two lifetime risk of developing cancer; for women, the risk is a little more than one in three. About 77 percent of all cancers are diagnosed in persons 55 years of age and older, but cancer is by no means an old person's malady. About one in four people who receive a cancer diagnosis is under the age of 55.

I am not among those who ascribe to the belief that cancer is some sort of gift, in any form. It is a terrible disease. But I do believe that we can learn from the people who have experienced it. And that is essentially what this book is about.

In the following pages, you will meet a diverse community of cancer patients, survivors, veterans, and their families, who offer a candid look at the way cancer has changed and shaped their lives. They share stories of discovery, adventure, and self-awareness that have occurred in spite of cancer in some cases and because of it in others.

Amy Nofziger of Denver, Colorado, describes her experience this way: "Cancer is just part of my life story," she says. "It's a chapter, but it's not the whole book. I will not let it define me." In the four years since her diagnosis, Amy has gone back to graduate school, received a job promotion, adopted a child, and traveled extensively.

After cancer, some people have climbed mountains, a literal and metaphorical accomplishment over their disease. Others have been sidelined by their illness, but still quietly reflect on the joy they find in life's most mundane moments.

As the stories and pictures shared in these pages will show you, life after cancer is not always simple or easy. But thankfully, it can be interesting, filled with celebrations, family vacations, obstacles, and even scars—all those things that ultimately define a life well lived.

Tara Parker-Pope writes about personal health for The New York Times *and is the editor of the paper's "Well" section.*

Sources for statistics:
American Cancer Society. *Cancer Facts & Figures 2012*. Atlanta: American Cancer Society; 2012.

American Cancer Society. *Cancer Treatment and Survivorship Facts & Figures 2012-2013*. Atlanta: American Cancer Society; 2012.

Acknowledgments

I would like to acknowledge the following people who made *Picture Your Life After Cancer* possible:

Aron Pilhofer and Andrew DeVigal, whose vision transformed a simple idea into a living, growing online community.

Jacqui Maher, Jon Huang, and Tom Jackson, whose expertise and patience were invaluable for making the online photo gallery possible.

Alice DuBois, Tara Parker-Pope, and Toby Bilanow, whose support was instrumental in getting this project off the ground and seeing it through to success.

Alex Ward, whose creative thinking helped to turn a digital photo gallery into something tangible and timeless.

And finally, thank you to L.T., who always knows how to dream big.

Karen Barrow
Editor

Introduction

By KAREN BARROW

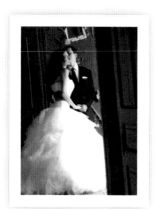

The New York Times asked readers who had survived cancer to send us their photos and answer the question, "How is your life different after cancer?" We had no idea what the reaction would be. It was the first time the health desk has tried anything like it. We were just hoping to get something, anything.

As usual, our readers did not disappoint. Within just a few hours, photos began to stream in, and by the end of the first week, we had more than a hundred images. And they kept coming, weeks and months later. Today, we have almost 1,000 beautiful, touching images.

We started the project because there is so much focus on treating and diagnosing cancer, but much less on its aftereffects. What happens to a person after agonizing amounts of time spent in doctors' waiting rooms? After grueling treatments that leave a person weak, nauseated, and spent? Does the stress of waiting for test results subside? Does the specter of cancer continue to haunt, or does normal life resume?

The images on our "Picture Your Life After Cancer" photo wall display the wide-ranging impact that cancer can have on a life in the months and years after the last doctor's appointment. The images

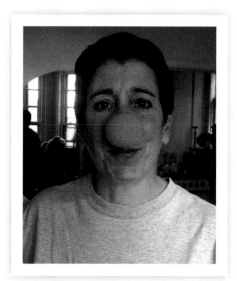

are more than snapshots and simple thoughts about life after a chronic disease; they are pictures of new adventures, grandchildren, vacations taken, marathons run, and lovely, smiling faces. They are also pictures of loss, confusion, and sadness. Surviving cancer doesn't always lead to a happy ending.

The photos are overwhelming in their variety, but it is the words that tell the full story. These are stories of hope, trepidation, concern, and renewal. These are tales of newfound love and redemption, words of deeply held beliefs, and sage advice.

Not all submissions came from someone whose story followed the expected narrative of diagnosis, treatment, and remission. Some were from individuals who never had cancer, but experienced the disease in another way. They may have helped a loved one through a cancer diagnosis or lost someone to the disease. Still other submissions came from those for whom a cure was not possible. For them, there was no life after cancer, only with.

We hosted a discussion on the photo collage on *The New York Times* Well blog for people to share their thoughts about the piece. There, Linnea Duff, a woman with stage IV lung cancer, explained why she participated even though she knows she won't have an "after cancer."

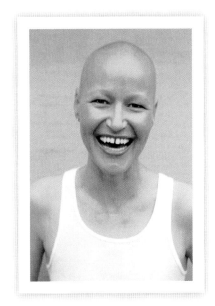

I proudly placed my photo on the wall, in part, as a reminder that there are many with cancer in my situation (or worse, those who have passed).

I find this pictorial wall, or collage, sad and amazing but also incredibly uplifting. Look at all those beautiful faces!

Cancer is awful and, for many, this disease both demands and takes away so much more than is fair. But, as traumatic as this experience may be, it bears telling. Sharing my own story is empowering; reading others' stories is a reminder that we are not alone.

As the producer of the "Picture Your Life After Cancer" project, I had the distinct honor of reading every single one of these submissions. And I was on the receiving end of the various reactions our readers had to the piece. It seemed that everyone had a different favorite, a different image or story that resonated most strongly. The most frequent comment I heard was how captivating the project was. You couldn't just click on one photo and leave; you kept flipping through the photos wondering what story the next one would tell.

Creating this book gave me the opportunity to reach out to those who had shared a piece of themselves on our Web site. Almost everyone who was asked to be included was happy to oblige. A few asked to update their submission to fill in the gaps from the last year or so.

Sadly, as the story goes with cancer, not everyone who posted his or her photo on the wall is still with us. And thus, in some cases, it was the parents, children, or spouses who replied to my requests with earnest disappointment that their loved one couldn't participate in the same way as the rest. So, I decided the truest picture of life after cancer would be to include the few who didn't get to complete their "after cancer" journey. They are here, too.

The "Picture Your Life After Cancer" photo collage continues to grow. We receive more submissions every week, as new people become part of the "after cancer" club. I hope that growth continues. And I hope that, through this project, both those who have just begun their tumultuous journey and those who have come out on the other side can take comfort in the fact that there is a large community of others out there who have tread the same path, fought the same demons, and felt the same way.

To see all of the images, or to add your photo to the collection, please visit www.nytimes.com/pictureyourlife.

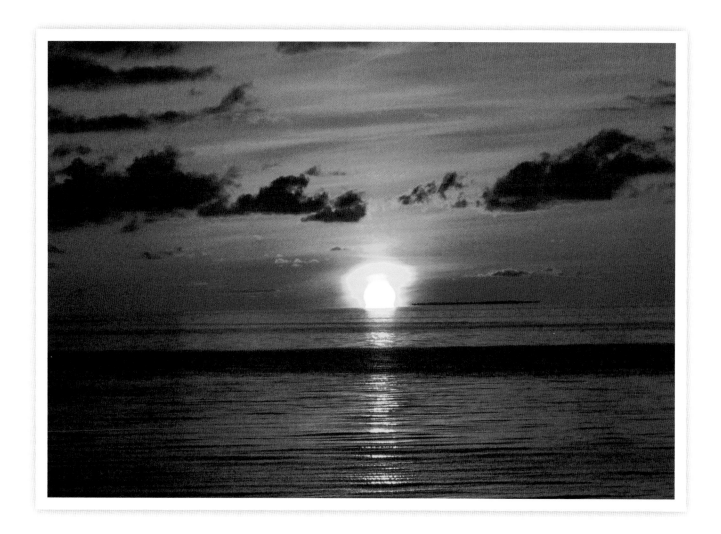

How is your life different after cancer?

Helene Strand

London, England

Life is different now because it is the only thing that matters after cancer. I don't worry about the small things anymore. I don't get annoyed by little problems that come my way. I love life, and I live it day by day. We can never know what will happen tomorrow, so make the most of today!

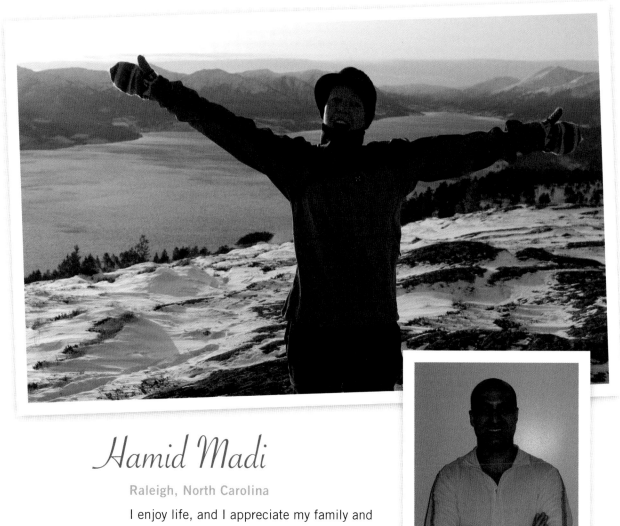

Hamid Madi

Raleigh, North Carolina

I enjoy life, and I appreciate my family and friends even more. Little things don't bother me as much, and the imminent birth of my first child is undoubtedly another reason I feel blessed to still be alive.

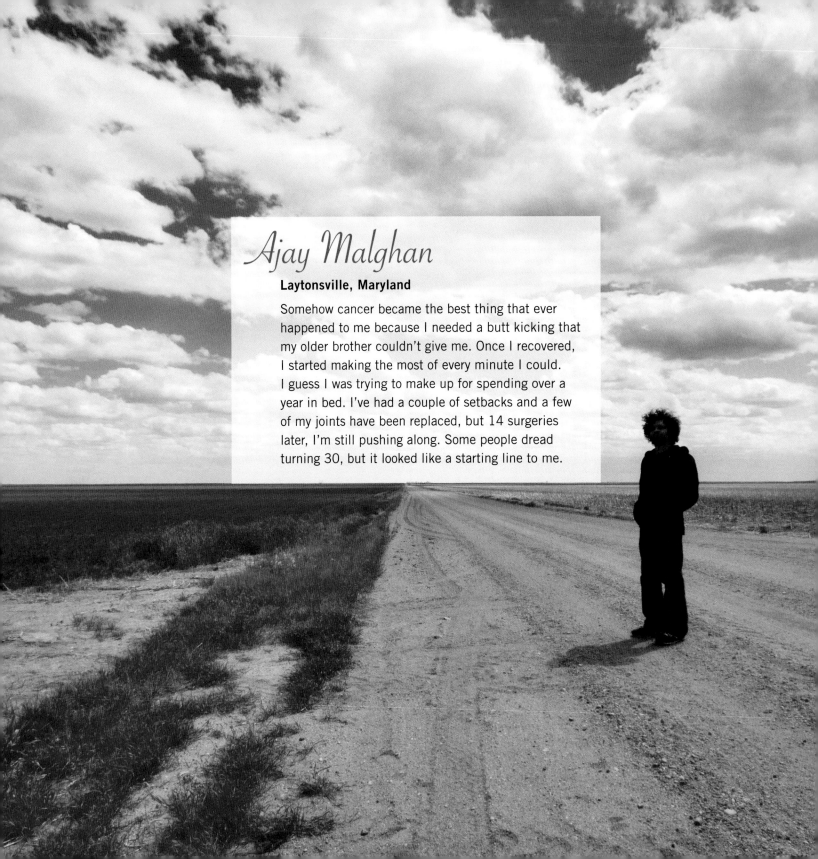

Ajay Malghan

Laytonsville, Maryland

Somehow cancer became the best thing that ever happened to me because I needed a butt kicking that my older brother couldn't give me. Once I recovered, I started making the most of every minute I could. I guess I was trying to make up for spending over a year in bed. I've had a couple of setbacks and a few of my joints have been replaced, but 14 surgeries later, I'm still pushing along. Some people dread turning 30, but it looked like a starting line to me.

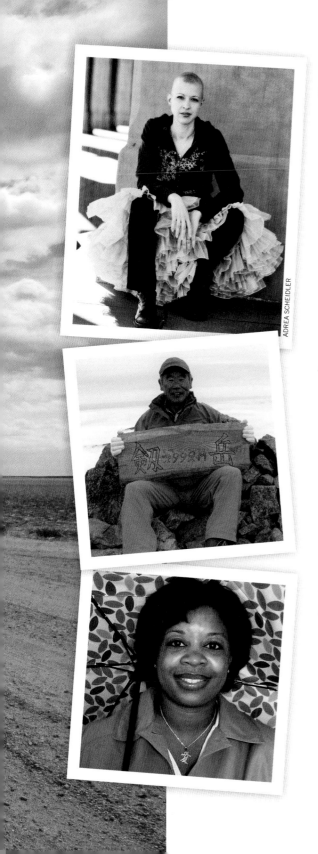

ADREA SCHEIDLER

Jennifer Gray

California

After cancer, I am vulnerable, soft, and emotional.
I am gritty, tough, brave, and bold.
I am afraid, and I am ready to kick some ass.

Cancer made me examine my deepest emotions and took me through my darkest times. Cancer has strengthened my relationships. Cancer has made me finally ready to go out there and live my life. I am not glad I had cancer, but, without it, I wouldn't be the *me* that I am today.

Kazuma Inoue

Osaka, Japan

I was sentenced to have two types of cancer just one month after I retired at the age of 61. Thanks to two different operations, I could come back to my daily life. After two years, I started again to climb mountains. I would like to climb all of the 100 famous mountains in Japan. So far, I have climbed 56. This photo was taken on my 56th mountain, Yarigatake.

Yodi Collins

Fairfax, Virginia

I "died" of cancer in 2004. Six months later, after a meticulous chemotherapy regimen, I was reborn into something remarkable. I have spent the years since then celebrating that giddy spring day. Today, I am love, hope, and joy—wisdom and strength.

Matt Garrison

Bath, New York

When I was preparing for a stem cell transplant to treat my leukemia, my wife, Cathy, bought this canoe. It is the best canoe in the world: a Minnesota II in graphite. Cathy said if I were to survive the transplant it would become my canoe, and we could keep paddling along together. Well, it's been almost six years now, and we have put over a thousand miles on the Min.

The thing is—mile by mile, year by year—it has become *our* boat, not just my boat. I guess that is what surviving is, getting back to *us*, not me.

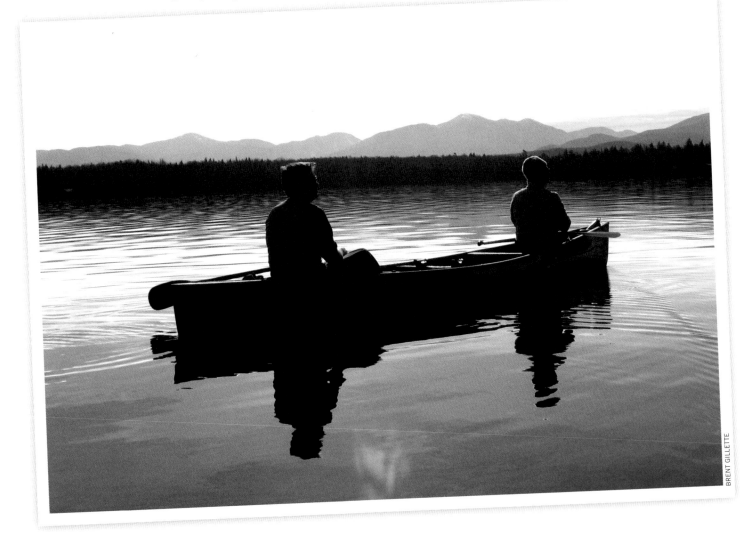

BRENT GILLETTE

Sarah Feather

Framingham, Massachusetts

Before I was diagnosed with cancer, I loved to sit around. Reading a book in a comfy chair with my cat was a perfect way to kill 8 or 10 hours. When my boys became toddlers and started running around, my sitting days ended, and I missed relaxing and being still.

Now that I have a legitimate excuse to be tired and sit down, I find that I don't want to sit so much anymore. I walk the dog. I cook dinner. I join committees. When I have the energy, and as my treatment schedule allows, I love to try new things that would have scared me before.

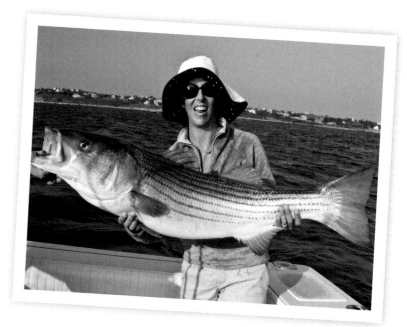

Although I still catch a healthy amount of good-natured ribbing from my family for my tendency to be a slug, we all know that I'm still here fighting, and I'm going to make the most of every minute.

Victoria Colliver Cautero

Berkeley, California

This photo is of me and my husband on our wedding day, just over three years after I finished chemotherapy and radiation for non-Hodgkin lymphoma. I've always said that if cancer is a gift, please direct me to the returns line. With that said, I prefer to concentrate on all the blessings I have in my life and not what cancer has taken from me. Here's to new hair, a loving partner, wonderful friends and family, and radiating in a whole different way.

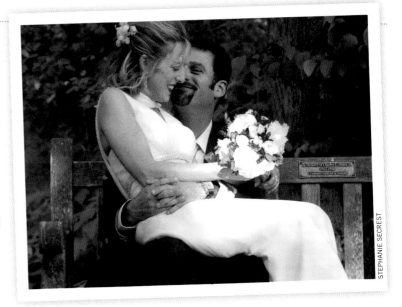

STEPHANIE SECREST

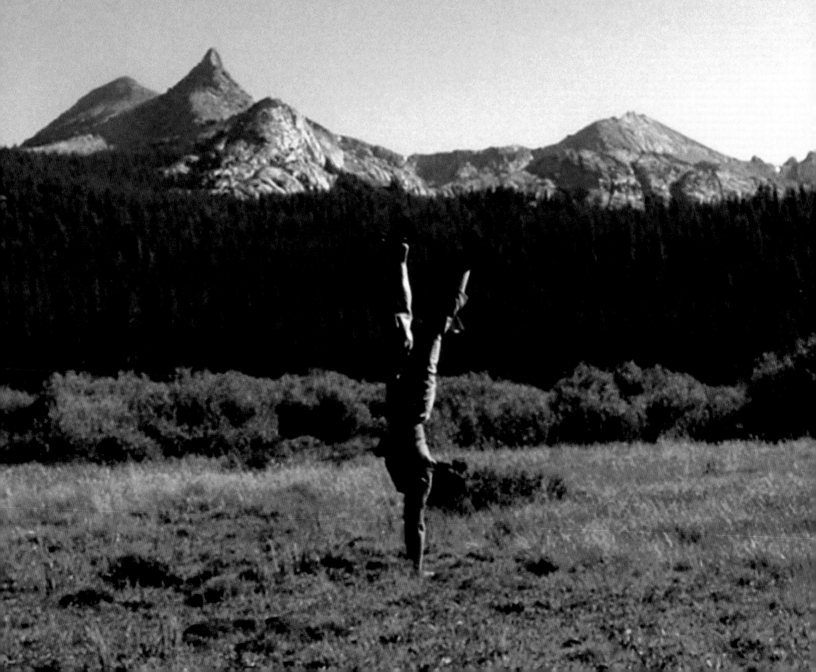

Zpora Perry

California

Sometimes life isn't that different, and I am still plodding through the day to day. But sometimes I am struck with a jolt of gratitude and joy that I am here, healthy, and happy. Doing handstands in a beautiful place can help me feel that way.

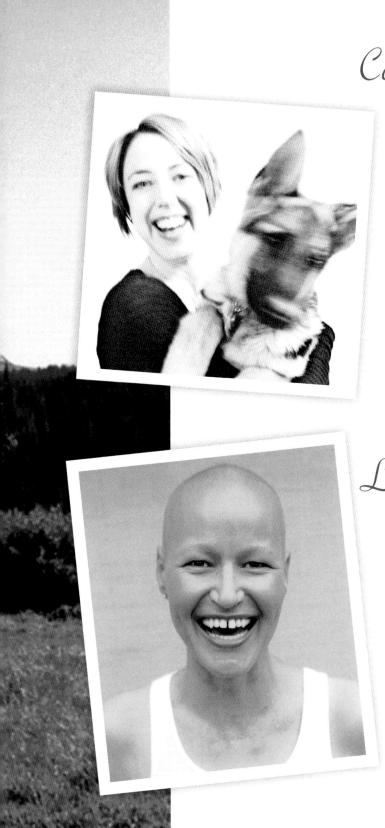

Cara Howell

Albuquerque, New Mexico

After four years of treatment for thyroid cancer, which included three rounds of radiation, a total thyroidectomy, and a partial neck dissection, I found my voice!

My diagnosis at age 27 occurred when I was trying to get pregnant. Instead of motherhood and the trappings of married life, my cancer experience exposed the unhappiness in my marriage and a lack of fulfillment in my life. Through the treatment process, I myself went through a kind of rebirth.

Today, I am starting over as a single woman in a new city and I couldn't be happier. I got a puppy and decided that play is often more important than work. Every single day, I try to love myself and those around me better. I adore the long, thin scar across my neck; it is beautiful for all these reasons and more.

Linnea Duff

Meredith, New Hampshire

For myself and many others with advanced cancer, we remain in treatment, and there is no life *after* cancer. Instead, I have had to learn to live *with* my cancer. Rather than calling myself a survivor, which would seem to suggest that the battle is over, I say that I am surviving. I just celebrated surviving five years since my cancer diagnosis.

As someone living with a terminal illness, I am acutely aware that each and every day is a gift, and I have learned to focus on the simple wonders of being alive.

Yarrott Benz

Los Angeles, California

As a high school teacher, one of my rules is transparency. I teach the fantastic subjects of art history and architecture, but I also teach something important by just being me—simply by example. My students learn that I grew up in the Tennessee of the Old South. They learn that I'm gay and comfortable with my sexuality. Recently, they also learned that I had a tumor on the base of my tongue from lymphoma—a story that announced itself with each word I mouthed.

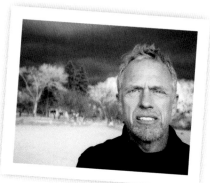

For three months, they watched my face turn red and my energy fluctuate from the chemotherapy and radiation. Then, as if breaking out of a cocoon, my voice shed its muffle and returned to its normal clarity. Perhaps watching their teacher face cancer openly will give my students something that will help them should they ever need it.

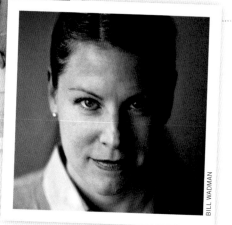

Susan Pohl

Berkeley, California

After cancer, my husband and I bonded in a unique way. He made the daily journey for my treatments and never missed a doctor's appointment. Although I loved him madly before the diagnosis, his presence has brought me laughter and balance during the darkest of times.

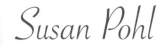

BILL WADMAN

Tisa DeForest

New York, New York

I feel grateful that I have to worry about taking my medication. On time. Every day. For the rest of my life.

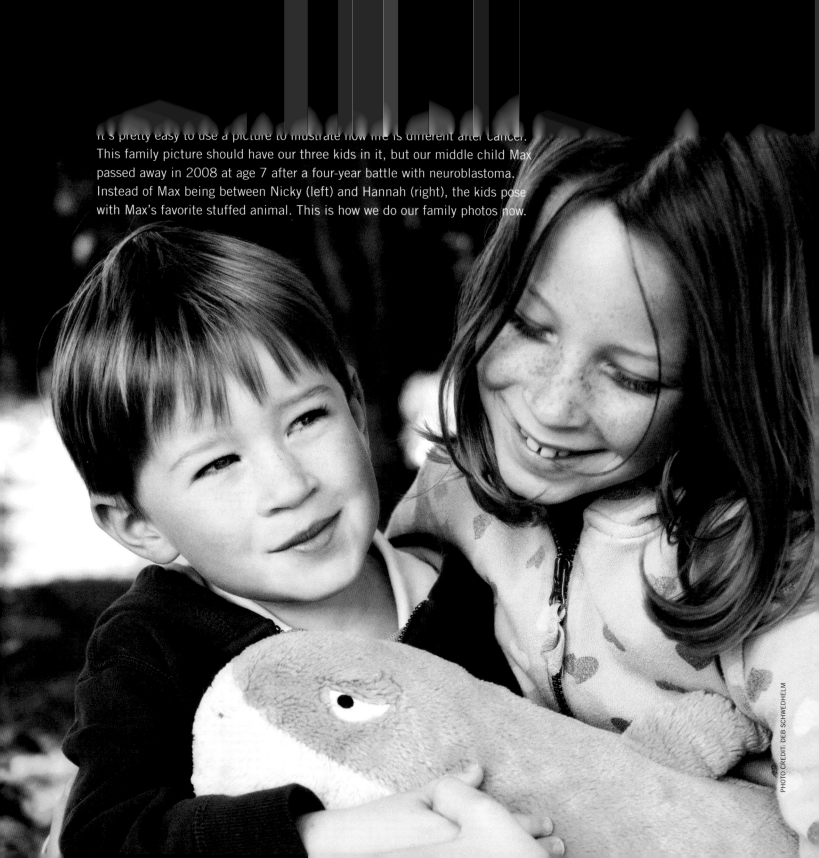

It's pretty easy to use a picture to illustrate how life is different after cancer. This family picture should have our three kids in it, but our middle child Max passed away in 2008 at age 7 after a four-year battle with neuroblastoma. Instead of Max being between Nicky (left) and Hannah (right), the kids pose with Max's favorite stuffed animal. This is how we do our family photos now.

Susan Moeller

Cape Cod, Massachusetts

When I first was diagnosed with stage III breast cancer, my older daughter said to me,
"You know, Mom, cancer sucks. But you're going to meet the most interesting people."
What an understatement, on both counts. I am lucky that cancer continues to broaden my world
more than it limits it. The strategy of finding out all I can about another person gives me focus
when I'm feeling self-conscious or worried about my own future.

Like other survivors, I'm grateful every day. This Christmas card reminds me that when all else fails
to banish my fears, dark humor and love help.

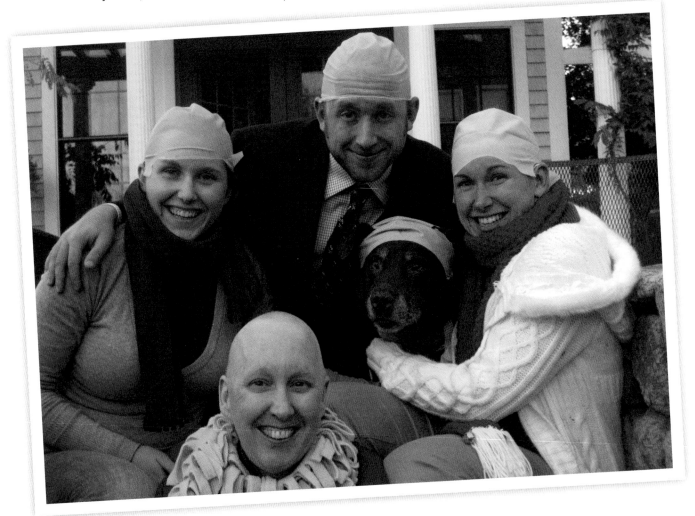

Sue Cloninger

New Orleans, Louisiana

It's been 14 months since my surgery for renal cell carcinoma. I was lucky because my cancer seems to have been isolated in my left kidney.

Am I different now? I hope so.

I try to not sweat the small stuff. I usually say what is on my mind and don't hold on to resentment. I also try to enjoy life since I know that all of our lives are finite. It makes me do things now rather than when I have the time.

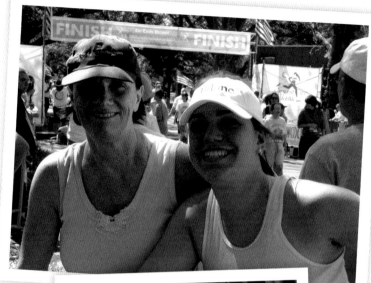

This picture was taken six weeks after my surgery while on a trip to my birthplace, New Orleans, where my daughter and I participated in a 10K race. After being an avid walker and runner for the past 23 years, this was the first race I completed. I figured if not now, then when? It was the beginning of the old me coming back to this world, where I hope to remain for a long time.

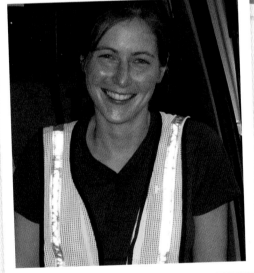

Mandy Stahre

Minnesota

Someone once said that having cancer is like being part of a club, but with one hell of an initiation. I was initiated at the age of 31 with a breast cancer diagnosis.

One week before my double mastectomy, I ran my eighth marathon. This picture was taken nine weeks later at the Ragnar Relay Great River Race. It was my first race after surgery. I ran with a different body, but I was running again.

Since the diagnosis, I've learned to appreciate the good days and allow myself to have bad days, too. I don't stress over little things. Most important, I take time out of each day for myself. I plan to keep running throughout the rest of the reconstructive surgeries, and maybe some day I'll make it into the 50 states marathon club. The initiation will be hard, but at least this time, it will be my decision.

Linda Misencik

Amherst, Ohio

I find that I don't worry about the small things as much anymore. It doesn't matter that my house isn't clean, or that I don't have the time to cook dinner every night. And my life doesn't revolve around my job anymore. I leave work at a decent hour so that I can live my life, train for triathlons, and spend time with my family. My husband and I are thinking of retiring early—to enjoy LIFE!

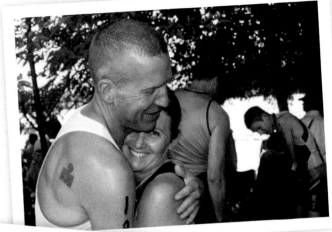

Linden Joesting

Lanikai, Hawaii

Life is more intense and sweeter—and more tiring than before. It's still so new to me that I don't quite know what to do, but I do know that I never want to go back.

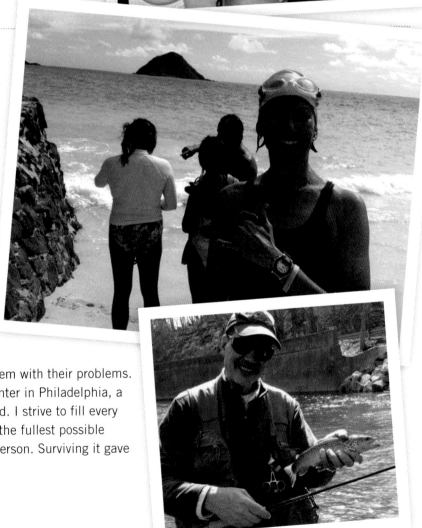

Bob Hesse

Jenkintown, Pennsylvania

I appreciate others more, and I try to help them with their problems. I am a volunteer at the Fox Chase Cancer Center in Philadelphia, a wonderful cancer hospital where I was treated. I strive to fill every minute and enjoy life, family, and friends to the fullest possible extent. Having cancer made me a different person. Surviving it gave me a better life.

Amy Nofziger

Denver, Colorado

Nobody on this planet gets out of here without a bag of crap, as I like to call it. We all carry around an invisible suitcase with our story in it. Cancer is no different. Cancer is just part of my life story. It's a chapter, but it's not the whole book. I will not let it define me.

It has been almost four years since I was diagnosed with ovarian cancer at the age of 30. Since then, I've climbed mountains, gone back to graduate school, received a promotion, adopted my youngest son, and traveled far and wide. Oh, and being bald isn't as bad as everyone says it is.

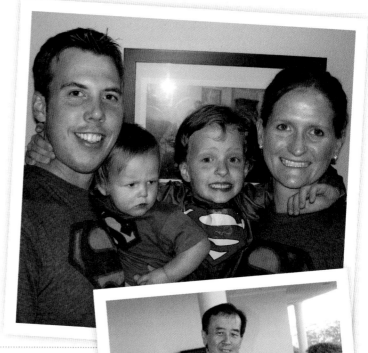

John Ishihara

Honolulu, Hawaii

After my cancer diagnosis in 2008, I retired. After I got better, I started to travel and went to Bali with my son in 2009. I've become more spiritual and aware of our connection to all things. I don't stress out anymore, and I try to accept whatever happens without judgment. If I don't like what has happened, I try to change it, but I don't judge.

Eileen Burkhart

Minnesota

We like to say that our lives have been enriched by having cancer, but that's just something we tell ourselves so we can go on despite our losses.

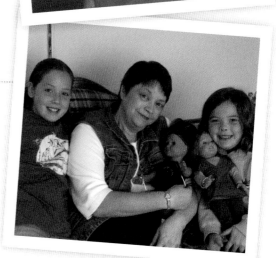

Rachel Oppenheimer

A Coruña, Spain

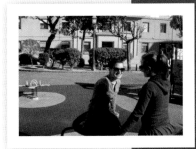

Life after cancer is great. I found a new sense of independence by moving to New York City just one week after my last chemotherapy session. I also traveled to Europe for spring break to visit two close friends who were studying in Spain.

This picture shows my college roommate, Florette, and me having fun at a playground in Galicia's beach city of A Coruña.

For me, life after cancer is vivid, and I feel awake in a way that I didn't before cancer. I feel the breezes more fully, see my loved ones more truly, and shed layers of my self-consciousness more easily.

Linda Updike

Grand Canyon, Arizona

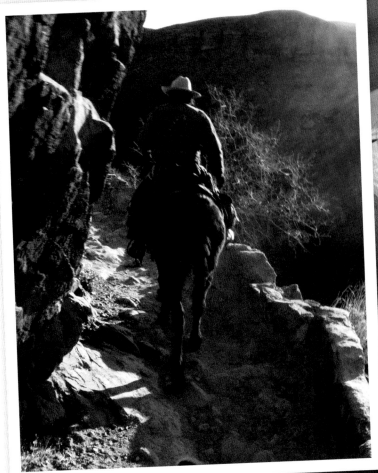

Every day, and I mean every single day, is a blessing after having cancer.

I have never been the type of person to have a cause, but as I lay in bed, unable to get up during chemotherapy, I decided that if I survived, my life needed to be about more than just me. I have become dedicated to doing all I can to find a cure for breast cancer. I started Team Grand Canyon at the Arizona Susan G. Komen 3-Day for the Cure. Last year we had just three members, but we raised over $16,000. This year, we hope to have 10 members and raise over $25,000.

I've learned to not sweat the small stuff, and if you, your friends, and your family are healthy, then everything else is truly just small stuff. Go Team Grand Canyon!

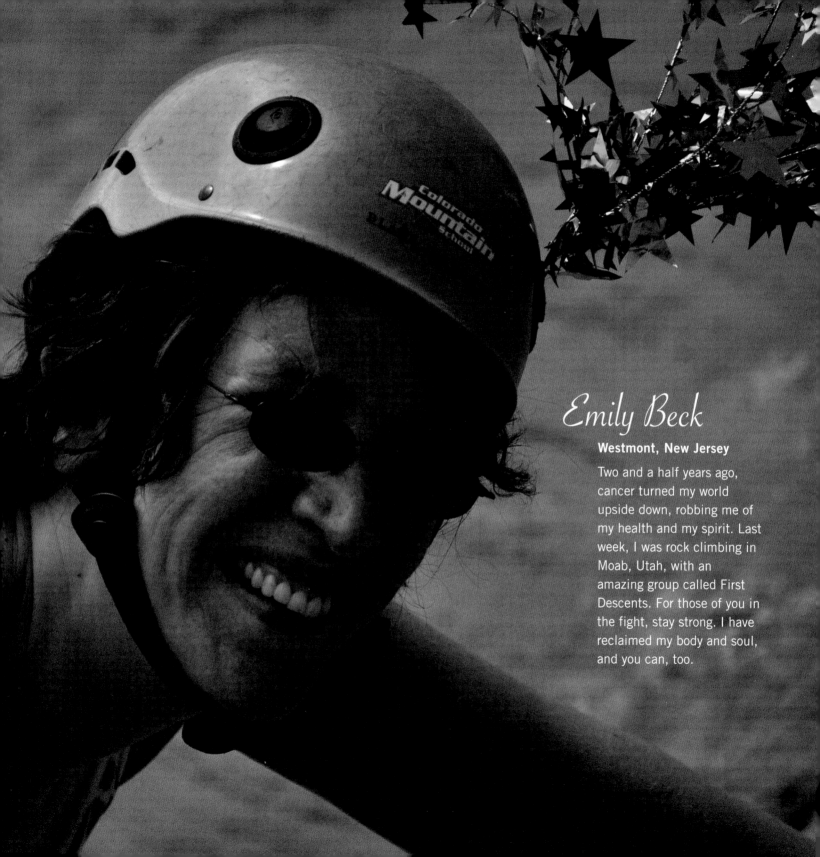

Emily Beck

Westmont, New Jersey

Two and a half years ago, cancer turned my world upside down, robbing me of my health and my spirit. Last week, I was rock climbing in Moab, Utah, with an amazing group called First Descents. For those of you in the fight, stay strong. I have reclaimed my body and soul, and you can, too.

Regina Falk

Keltern, Germany

As a nonsmoker and otherwise healthy person, breast cancer had nothing to do with me—until the summer of 2007. It took me quite a while to accept that nothing would be the same after that. The love and support of my husband and two children helped me find a new normal with more ups and downs than before. Today, I feel stronger than ever. I am trying to learn that every single day is something special and that the things I'd love to do should be done now, not later.

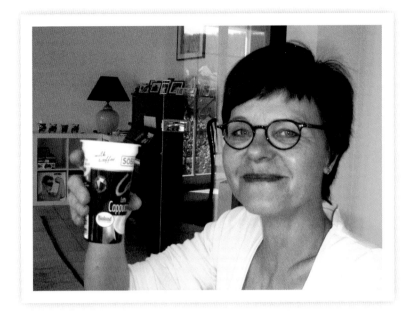

G. Wayne Curtis

Lee's Ferry, Arizona

My kidney cancer was discovered last year in what the doctors called an "accidental finding" during a CT scan taken for other reasons. Thanks to that scan, and several doctors, my life was saved.

How is my life different? I now take religion seriously. It was not a fortunate accident, but the hand of God. When I was a boy in Georgia, I often saw signs nailed up on trees by the side of the road that said, "Are you ready to meet your God?" Well, I never was before, but I am now. It is sobering because I have begun to see eternity in the distance, as one sees the sun when clouds begin to dissipate.

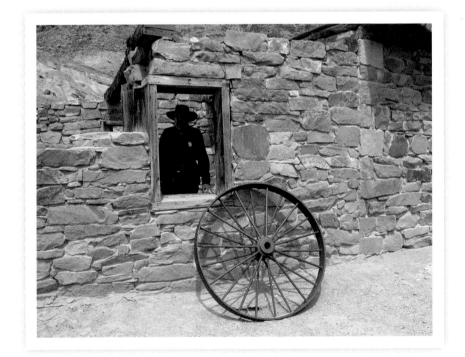

Anthony Baccaro

Big Pine Key, Florida

I've had cancer twice—first, when I was 17 and again, a few years ago. I freely admit that having cancer when I was young made a lasting impression on me. Cancer made my life exceedingly challenging at a very impressionable time of life.

Much later, like an unexpected gift, it left me with an overwhelming sense of wonder at all the potential for passion in this life—passion that too often doesn't get to be fully experienced because we're too occupied by the necessities of making our way through life. And yet, life is indifferent and impartial. It continuously offers rebirth, yet frames that rebirth around a limited band of time. I believe the raw beauty of nature is the ultimate guardian of that time.

I've chosen a beautiful sunset for my picture. A sunset isn't only an ending; the sun also rises!

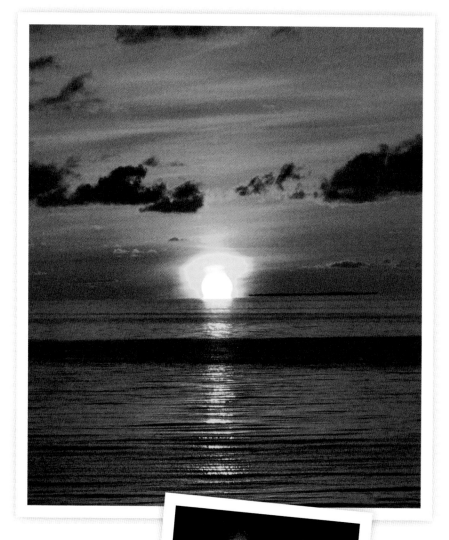

Adriana Rubio

Los Angeles, California

This picture is of my dad, Vince Rubio, dancing at his 50th birthday party. He was almost three years cancer free on the day this picture was taken.

Just a few weeks ago, we found out his cancer has returned. We are praying and hopeful. We can't wait to celebrate like this when he beats it again!

Pat Curry

Rochester, New York

A diagnosis of kidney cancer in April 2007 motivated me to get busy living. I returned to college to pursue a second degree, a B.F.A. in drawing, which was a dream I'd been saving for old age. I also took to exercise and community service. Now, my husband and I train each summer for an annual fundraising bicycle ride in September. I've been very open about my cancer journey and thankful for the support and encouragement of my family, friends, physicians, and coworkers, as well as a lot of strangers along the way.

I hope a lot more now. I make it a point to reach out to those in my life who have a new cancer diagnosis. My spirit felt vulnerable when I got the news, but is now stronger than ever. Hope, laughter, and encouragement are the best tools in surviving cancer!

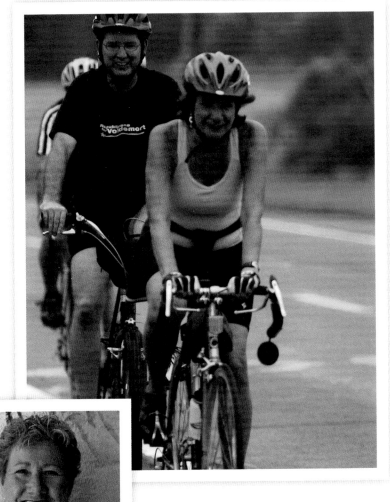

Ruth Cole Spies

Punta Gorda, Florida

It's me with curly hair! I've become a cancer activist. We must support cancer research so our grandchildren and their children will never have to fear a diagnosis of cancer. I try to do what I can to raise cancer awareness and promote the search for a cure in my column for the local newspaper.

Knowing that there was an 87 percent chance that chemotherapy would cause the loss of all my body hair, I opted to shave my head just after my first chemotherapy infusion. Being bald was an emotionally and physically freeing experience. I no longer had to worry about spending too much time styling my hair—I saved a ton of money on hair care products during my nearly eight months of "billiard ballism"!

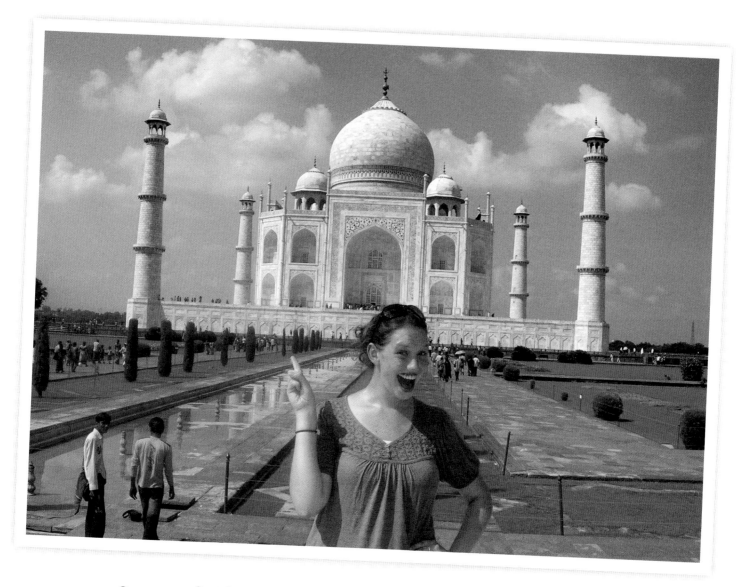

Laura Werner

St. Paul, Minnesota

I am more adventurous now. Every time a new opportunity presents itself, instead of second guessing and wondering whether I can do it or not, I go for it! I didn't really have that in me before becoming a cancer survivor. I am thankful for the newfound urgency that surviving cancer has given my life.

Alexa Landsman

Charlotte, North Carolina

I'm no longer afraid of cancer. I beat it! Just three weeks after my surgery last summer, I headed off to Europe to study abroad. I went to England to study, but I also got to visit Paris on the weekend. It was one of the best trips of my life. At first, I was a little reluctant to go, but the doctors told me I would be fine. The trip took my mind off the cancer. A month later, I had my radiation treatment.

Cancer can't stop me! To my friend (shown left), thank you for supporting me through the worst and best parts of my life!

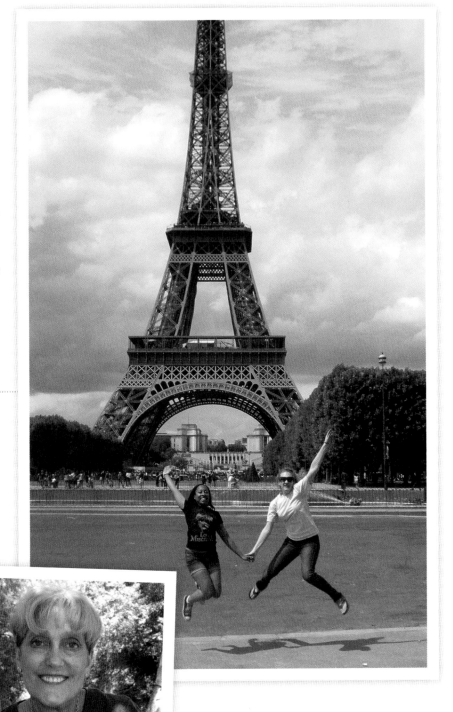

Catherine Cook

California

I had breast cancer in 1999. That year included my diagnosis, lumpectomy, and treatment. It was a wake-up call. Since then, I try to do the things I want to do. I am not saving money for any specific reason. When I have extra money, I spend it on things I want to do— charities or whatever. I am more aware that we are really mortal.

Donna Detwiler

North Lima, Ohio

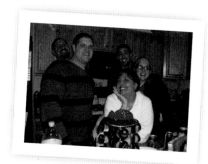

I am a seven-year survivor of multiple myeloma. I underwent a stem cell transplant two years ago, and I am now doing well.

Cancer has changed my life in many ways. I am a strong advocate for cancer patients, and I have started a local support group. I see how precious life and family are, and I am living every day to the fullest. I am a stronger person now with a stronger faith in God. That is the blessing in all of this, I guess. Blessings to all!

Jennifer Elizabeth Sica

Farmingdale, New York

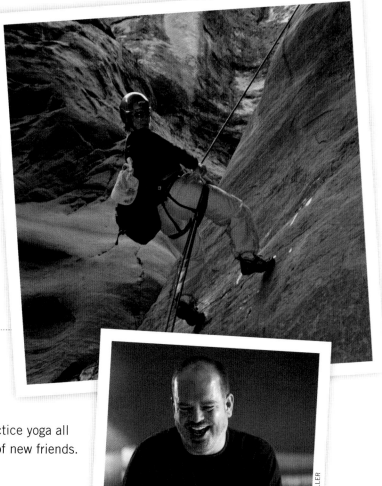

Life after cancer is special. Who knew that cancer could be such a blessing? I am thriving in the new me, the person who takes chances and is living life to the fullest.

I will take that path less traveled and enjoy making memories with every breath in my body. I laugh more. I appreciate the little things in life that I would have formerly ignored. I stopped sweating the small stuff. Life is good.

Jeff Paup

Seattle, Washington

Except for the cancer, my life is much better. I practice yoga all the time. I give and get massages. I've made a lot of new friends. I travel more and am much more adventuresome.

I am able to separate the important things from the chaff.

STEVEN MILLER

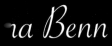

ᴍa Benn

cago, Illinois

er will I . . .

Spend an entire day inside.

Go for a week without exercise.

Go a day without telling my family that I love them.

Forget to be thankful.

Lose my voice.

Forget what it's like to struggle with a flight of stairs.

Forget what it feels like to be betrayed by my body.

Forget what it feels like to be pitied.

Forget what having no immune system feels like.

Forget the power of the mind.

Pretend to be a cancer expert.

Forget to breathe.

Forget life's fragility.

Forget what God feels like.

Forget that in order to experience today, I need to live
in this moment.

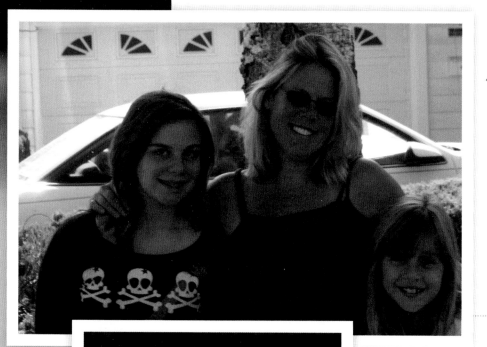

KayDee Stevens
California

I live every moment like I am going to die. I take advantage of every moment and smile much more. I don't wake up in the middle of the night scared to death that I have cancer anymore. I know who my friends are, and I bless them every day.

Lynda A. Levy
Los Angeles, California

My diagnosis freed me to be the person I was meant to be. I always wanted to perform the "Great American Songbook" and work with wonderful musicians. I finally did it! I had many gigs around my town, my favorite being The Gardenia Supperclub. So now, I am the "singing psychotherapist" and I love every moment of both careers, on and off the stage.

My life is rich and full with six grandchildren. My husband, Stan, and I have been married for 47 years. I am doing everything I've ever wanted to do. I'm inspired by others, and my hope is that I can inspire others, too.

Listen to your heart.

Maria Virginia Sanchez

New York

I made it!

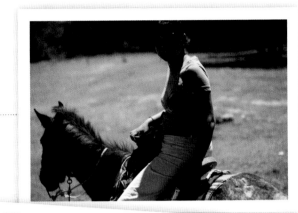

Loren Brill

New York, New York

Life is very different after cancer. I look at my quality of life, health, and nutrition very differently. After recovering from Hodgkin disease four years ago, I stopped eating refined, processed, or unnatural foods. But even with my insatiable sweet tooth, I could not find baked goods that were not made from refined ingredients. So, I started baking, using only all-natural, wholesome ingredients. It's a myth that you can't make unbelievably delicious treats with 100 percent whole grains, no refined sugars, and no dairy!

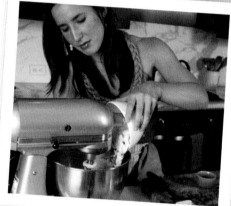

After years of friends and family taste testing, and much recipe tweaking, I came up with recipes for cookies and brownies that people just loved. And Sweet Loren's was born. Now, I am making it easier to live a deliciously healthy lifestyle.

Virginia McCabe

New Jersey

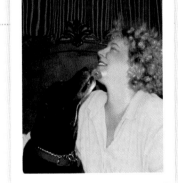

Life has been hard for me after breast cancer. I lost both breasts to save my life, but I am very grateful for so many things now. I am quieter, more contemplative, and feel emotions more deeply. I feel pain almost every hour of every day from the side effects of chemotherapy. One day the pain may go away. So I am hopeful.

My whole life has changed. I used to be extroverted, but now it is a chore to do even small things. I have turned to music and art to find joy and meaning in my life. I am still alive, and where there is life, there is hope. I have never given up hope.

I worry about other women who do not have insurance. I think about them. Where will their hope come from?

Martha Straus

Brattleboro, Vermont

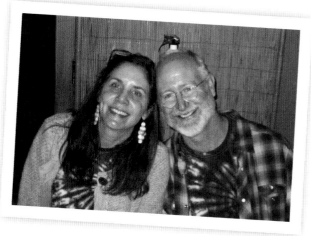

Within days of being diagnosed, I met Mike, the loveliest man I have ever known. Our early dates, before we'd even been to the movies, included trips to the hospital. Still, he was completely unfazed, even when the nurse gave him books with titles such as *When the Woman You Love Has Breast Cancer.*

Before I got sick, I was an anxious person. I worried about all kinds of things. Then, the worst thing actually happened. But falling in love at the same time that I began dealing with cancer provided me with a new life strategy. I now fret infrequently—everything else is paltry in comparison.

I feel joyful every day. In this photo, we are on our first post-cancer trip to California at a San Francisco theme party where everyone wore matching shirts!

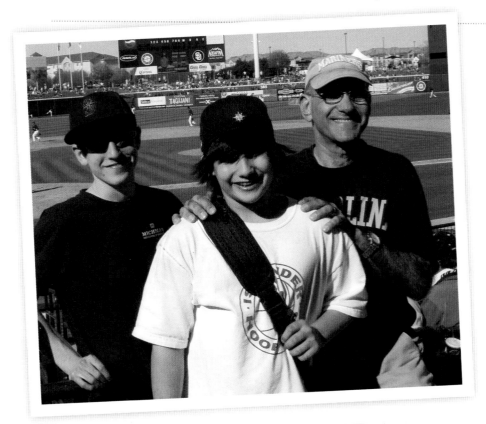

Andrew Schorr

Seattle, Washington

Fourteen years after being diagnosed with chronic lymphocytic leukemia and 10 years after participating in a phase II clinical trial, I remain in "molecular remission" and can celebrate life with my three kids. My youngest, Eitan (shown in front), will have his bar mitzvah soon. He is the miracle baby we never would have had if our specialist had not encouraged us. So now I am leukemia free, and he is about to be a man in the Jewish religion. Cool!

Heather Swift

San Mateo, California

Ithaca, New York

As a young-adult survivor, I have dedicated my life after cancer to supporting, educating, and advocating for the special needs of the 15- to 40-year-old population.

I find love and grace in every day despite physical pain, the side effects of treatment, and the ever-present possibility of recurrence. I have challenged myself in ways that I never would have before cancer—physically, intellectually, and emotionally.

I've given myself permission to grieve, acknowledge my losses, experience my emotions fully, and find joy in everything—including the hardships—while working to provide that space for others. I love deeply, live passionately, and look for the beauty in each moment, each day.

Jana-Lynn Kam

San Mateo, California

My goal in life is to do what makes me happy. I eat delicious foods that tickle my taste buds— like ice cream!

I exercise and appreciate the strength in my body. I have two 5Ks coming up. I have traveled to Belize and parts of Africa and seen the world.

I cherish my friends and family who have given me their never-ending support and love.

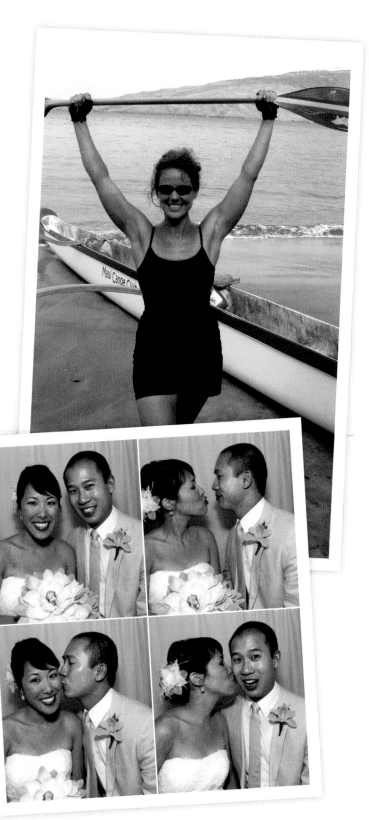

Julie Yamamoto

Olympia, Washington

The hair loss triggered a lot of play with my identity. Here, I take on Uncle Fester.

Cancer has shifted my focus. I'm spending more time connecting with friends and ignoring the little stuff. I'm trying to figure out where I'm headed and trying to be more open to flow and change, rather than digging in my heels. I feel a strong need for major changes in the work I do and with whom I spend time, and in knowing which battles are worth fighting.

I was doing much of this reflection and questioning many midlife issues before the cancer, but my diagnosis accelerated the process.

Humor is a staple of my experience. Without it, things would be too bleak.

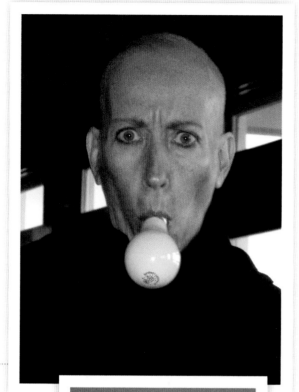

Hillary Hassink

Oklahoma

On July 21, 2010, I was diagnosed with stage II Hodgkin disease. After I was diagnosed, I thought my life was over. I had to withdraw from my college's nursing program so that I could undergo chemotherapy. I was devastated.

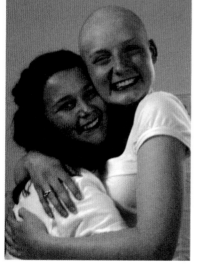

But then, a cancer survivor told me, "Cancer is 100 percent attitude." Now that I am done with my treatments, I could not agree more. Cancer does not mean death, and my life is not over. I am passing over a little bump in the road. When I return to school, this entire experience will only make me a better nurse. I know what it feels like to be sick, weak, and poked a million times like a human pincushion.

After I am done with chemotherapy, I will return to college and continue on my path to become an amazing nurse with extreme care and love.

Maggie Stenz

Brooklyn, New York

I have an implant in my right breast, so it doesn't look or feel exactly like my natural left breast. But that doesn't stop me from working out at the gym, playing softball, or playing with my kids. I don't know if I've fully sorted through the experiences of the past few years. My diagnosis in May 2009 was followed by three surgeries that summer. But I am not letting my status as a survivor define who I am or what I do.

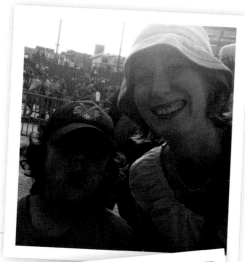

Michael J. Keegan

Chicago, Illinois

After having undergone a successful radical prostatectomy, I have both pain and residual issues. But knowing that I am still cancer free after several years and do not need radiation or chemotherapy has liberated me.

I take my passport to work with me and book trips overseas whenever I want. I buy whatever I want on Michigan Avenue, and I say and do whatever I please. I have been liberated from the inhibitions that held me back prior to surgery and motivated by my awareness of life's brevity and precious nature.

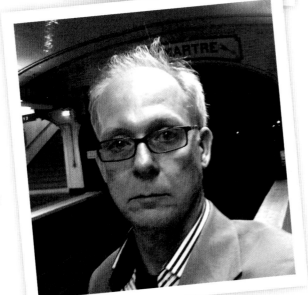

Donovan Bailey

Jacksonville, Florida

Every time I get sick, Mommy and Daddy and my sisters think the cancer has come back. My cancer has about a 40 percent cure rate. I try to play like a normal kid, but I get hurt and sick easier than other kids my age. Please help fight childhood cancers!

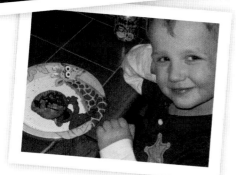

Debra Thompkins

Madison, Wisconsin

I was diagnosed with stage IIIB breast cancer when my daughter, Natasha, was in kindergarten. She gave me the strength to endure a solid year of treatment. She will be entering the fourth grade this year, and I feel great. I take the time to enjoy life much more now than before cancer, when the reality of my own mortality was so abruptly thrown at me.

A friend shared the following sayings with me, and I live by these words every day:

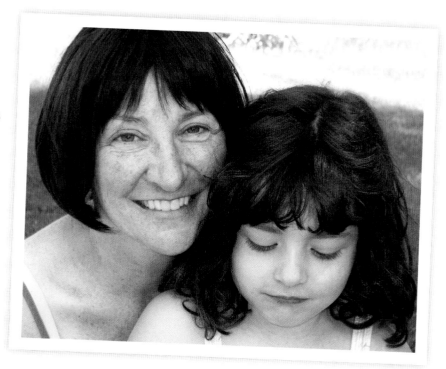

"What can one do? Go home, love your children, try not to bicker, eat well, walk in the rain, feel the sun on your face, and laugh loud and often, as much as possible, and especially at yourself."

"The antidote to death is not poetry, drama, miracle drugs, or a roomful of technical expertise and good intentions. The antidote to death is life."

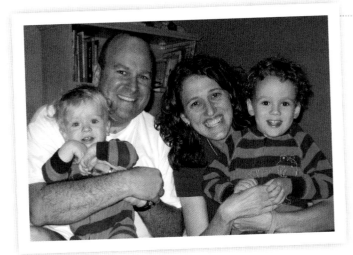

Dianne Caridi

Gainesville, Florida

I am a 22-month survivor of lung cancer with two young kids. I have never smoked. I can't say that I am *after* cancer, but I can say that I am living my life *with* cancer. I am happy to be here every day, even when life seems extra hard. I wouldn't want to miss a single minute with my two children, Joey and Anthony, and my husband, Joe.

Alison McManus

Seattle, Washington

No one expects to be diagnosed with cancer. At age 24, it made my life seem very short. Time was going by so fast and there were so many things I hadn't gotten to yet. After having my thyroid taken out, and with it the follicular carcinoma, I feel like I am a more engaged participant in my own life.

Time stretches into memories when we are learning new things. Luckily, there is a lot to learn and relearn, so that time may slowly drift by. Fast or slow, I let it be with no regrets.

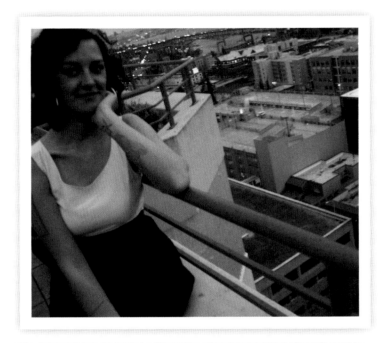

Danny D. Yeung

San Francisco, California

I get out of bed before dawn and show up at the tennis court or golf course before most of the other players. All the time, I hear myself saying to my tennis and golf buddies, "We are very lucky. What a wonderful day."

I try to look up every word that I don't know using my iPhone dictionary. I want to learn to write like my daughter, the journalist. I want to live my best life from now on.

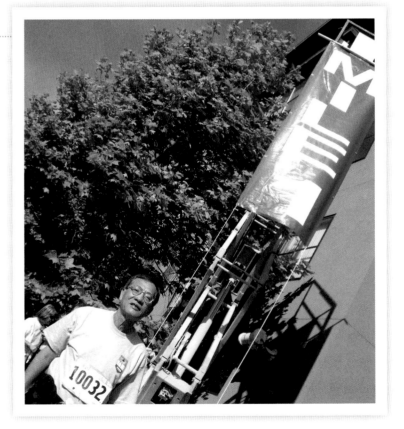

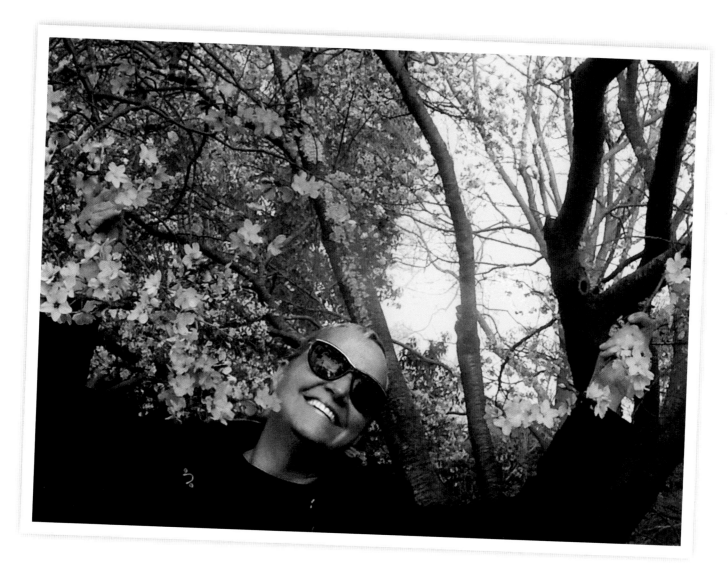

Deborah DeFranco

New Jersey

I am terrified of dying. I feel vulnerable. The big cancer institute missed my cancer. I no longer feel attractive. I lost my mojo. I have complications from the medications. My current position is seeing doctors—a lot of doctors. I graduated first in my class, but now I can't think like I used to. I lost my light. My world has gotten very small.

Gena Calderon

Hermosa Beach, California

I've always appreciated my life after fighting an autoimmune disorder that was treated with chemotherapy 21 years ago. But after surviving stage IV breast cancer, I have an even deeper appreciation for life.

Every day is a good day, rain or shine. There is beauty in everything if I look with both eyes open. I have a huge appetite for life, and I feel fearless. I try and do things I would never have done before.

The greatest gift has been the new perspective my husband has: to not sweat the small stuff. He's now ready to join me and experience life to its fullest. We share our lives with a greater sense of purpose. We'll be going skydiving soon.

I woke up breathing, so life is good.

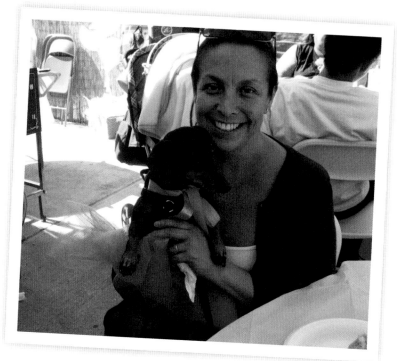

Heike Bill

Jakarta, Indonesia

My connection to myself has changed, and so has everything else. Today, I have conscious access to my inner resources. I accept what is: the flow of life, constant change, the motion inside me. I have choices, and that realization still moves me. I understand that I need to stay connected to feel alive. Connecting with another human being is, for me, one of the most beautiful and touching experiences.

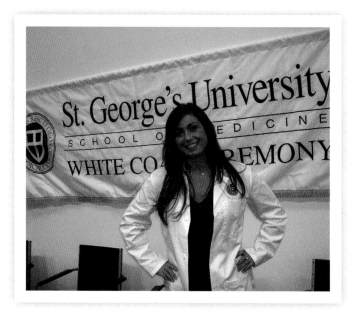

Julia Brockway

Staten Island, New York

Before cancer, I wanted to be a doctor. During treatment, I aspired to be like *my* doctors. Fifteen years after cancer, I am halfway to becoming a doctor.

Life is no different—it's the same blessing of ups and downs and good and bad it always has been. Cancer just gave life purpose.

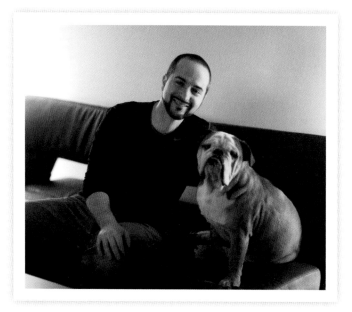

Jeff Derringer

Brooklyn, New York

I am more focused on my creative output than I was before I got sick. I am also trying to live more in the moment and in line with my priorities. However, it is a daily struggle to live with this level of fear and anxiety about my health, which was not a part of my experience before cancer. It's the yin and the yang; I'm appreciative of the moment, but also conscious of how few moments there actually are to be had.

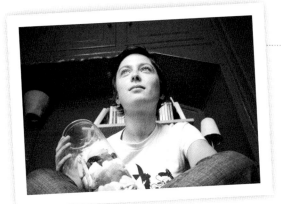

Julie Lyonnard

Washington, District of Columbia

I just see physicians more often than I used to.

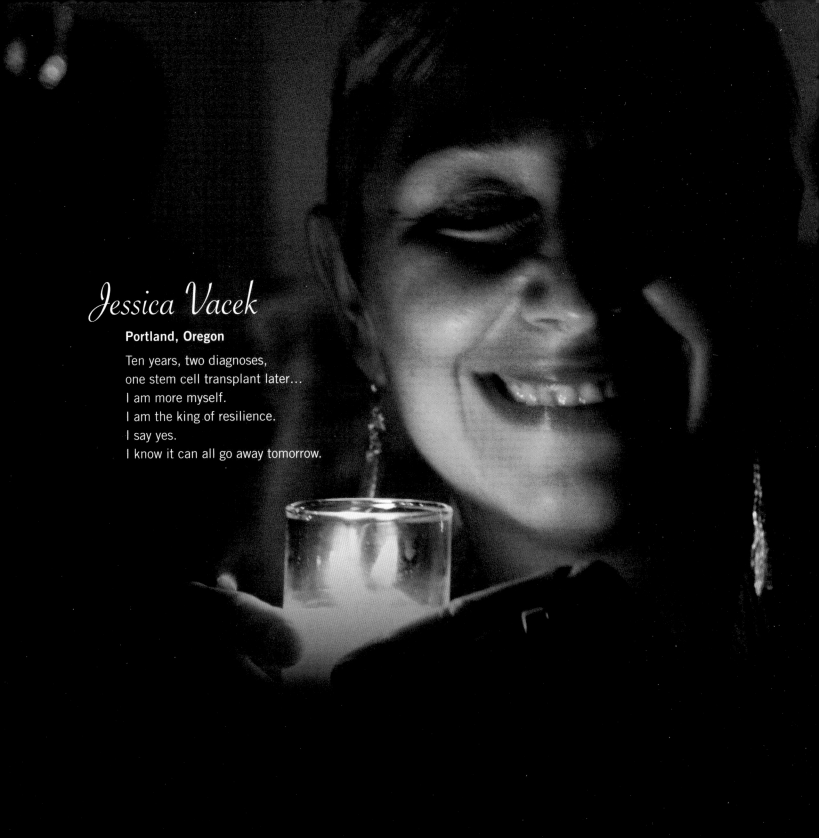

Jessica Vacek

Portland, Oregon

Ten years, two diagnoses,
one stem cell transplant later...
I am more myself.
I am the king of resilience.
I say yes.
I know it can all go away tomorrow.

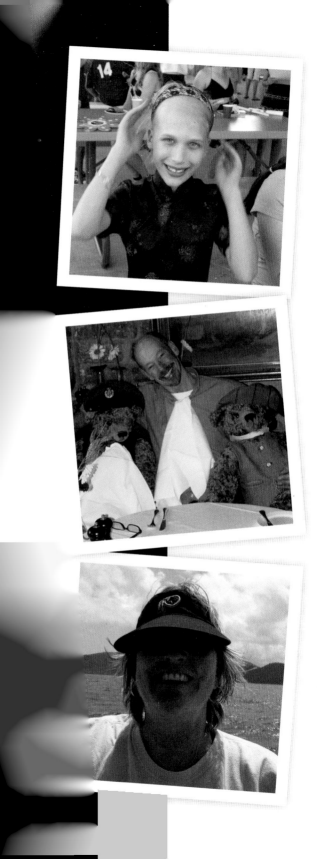

Karla Knudson

Kansas

My daughter, Annika, was diagnosed with Burkitt lymphoma at age 11. By age 12, she was a survivor. Now, she lives her life in the wake of cancer. She has an understanding of the fragility and preciousness of life. She is joyous and thankful. Her prognosis for long-term survival is good. But to even have to think about the chance of relapse is pretty heavy stuff for a kid. Annika knows several children who have died, and she has seen her friends relapse. Childhood cancer will always be with her, but she faces each day smiling, with her heart full of love and hope.

Thom Weyand

Oxfordshire, England

I'll never be able to answer the question: Why am I still here when others are not? How did I navigate the stormy waters of HIV and AIDS for the better part of a quarter century? How did I survive two occurrences of non-Hodgkin lymphoma (NHL) within less than a year? How did I get past being the 11th patient in the City of Hope stem cell transplant protocol for people with HIV and NHL?

These don't really seem like such important questions now. I am on the eve of what the medical community refers to as a clinically significant fifth anniversary of remission; I am just blessed to be able to keep on truckin'.

Lynne Streeper

St. Thomas, U.S. Virgin Islands

Every day is a gift, and I appreciate everything so much more! Colors are more vivid, moments are more meaningful, and I am so blessed and thankful.

Wendy Sorrell

Olympia, Washington

I savor each moment just a little bit more. Mine was an aggressive form of breast cancer, so I went through chemotherapy and radiation. Now, I feel excellent.

Good luck to all of you!

Naomi Brown

Sugar Land, Texas

After chemo, radiation, and surgery, and then losing my husband of 30 years to brain cancer, I have dedicated myself to a life of fitness. Being a cyclist and riding thousands of miles over the past three years has transformed me from a puny, middle-aged woman to a superstar athlete— at least to me. I have ridden all over the United States and France, even riding up the famous Col du Tourmalet, which is one of the stages of the Tour de France. Life is good.

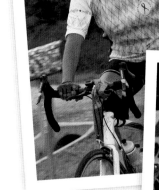

Amy Dodson

Sahuarita, Arizona

I lost my leg and my lung to undifferentiated sarcoma 25 years ago. What I got in exchange was perspective. I wouldn't trade my journey for anything.

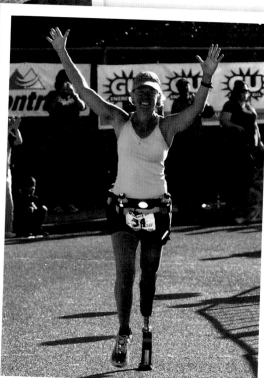

Musa Mayer

New York, New York

My breast cancer diagnosis 21 years ago took my life in a whole new direction. Having cancer inspired me to become a trained advocate and to write three books and numerous articles about cancer.

I work on behalf of women with metastatic breast cancer. My interest is in research and drug development, and I serve as a patient representative with the F.D.A. on many steering committees and with data monitoring boards for clinical trials and other studies. In representing patients, I take into account not only my own experiences, but those of the many women living with advanced breast cancer. While there is reason to hope, research can be encumbered by many perverse incentives. Trained advocates like me represent crucial voices around the table where decisions are made!

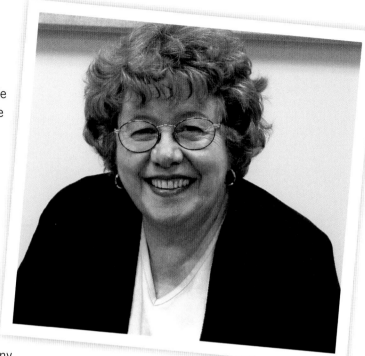

Nancy Bruning

New York, New York

I've lived half of my life after cancer, so it's hard to remember life before. One thing is for sure, though: my innocence is gone. I know that bad things can happen to good people, and they do.

After cancer, I switched to writing books about health and wellness. My master's degree in public health and my career as a lifestyle coach are at opposite ends of the spectrum—trying to help people be healthier and enjoy life as much as possible.

In this photo, I'm leading a "fitness al fresco" class at my local park, and three ladies in saris showed up! Who knows what is around the corner? Who knows how much time any of us has left, cancer or not?

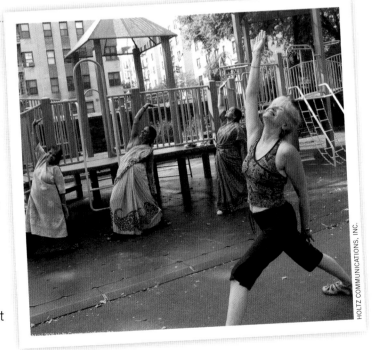

HOLTZ COMMUNICATIONS, INC.

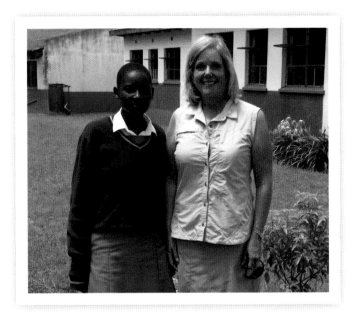

Kris McKinney

Denver, Colorado

I traveled to Africa, which has been a lifelong dream! I got to meet the orphans in Swaziland that we had been sponsoring for several years. I know now how fragile life is. When opportunities arise, you should take advantage of them. Don't keep waiting to follow your dreams and find your purpose. As some say, the curse of the cure is finding your meaning in life. Live!

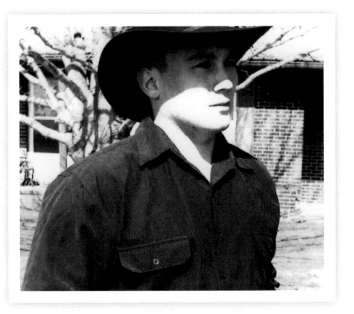

Jason Flatt

Cookeville, Tennessee

Life is better. It has taught me to think on my feet. I was 10 when I was diagnosed with brain cancer, so I was not that old. After cancer is when things started to happen.

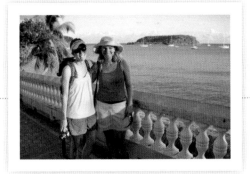

Elizabeth Dols

West Chester, Pennsylvania

I don't have an "after cancer," I have a "with cancer." I've been in treatment for lung cancer for four and a half years. Now, I am taking a new drug and participating in a clinical trial. I try to fill my life with the people I care about, visit the places that make me happy, and fill my days with normal activity. For me, it is all about hope.

Erik Marrero

Sewell, New Jersey

I appreciate my family more. I had kidney cancer in 1997, prostate cancer in 2002, and a recurrence of prostate cancer in 2005. My oncologist recommended Mindfulness-Based Stress Reduction (MBSR) to deal with the stress and side effects of cancer and treatment. MBSR teaches meditation and simple yoga to help you cope.* This was my introduction to yoga. Now, I teach yoga and the mindfulness that comes with its practice. Without the return of my cancer, I would not be practicing or teaching yoga today.

*For a complete discussion of mindfulness and other complementary therapies, see the American Cancer Society Complete Guide to Complementary and Alternative Therapies, or visit cancer.org.

Amanda Pope

Washington, D.C.

A diagnosis of thyroid cancer in early 2009 opened up my world and gave me a new direction in life. I started a young adult cancer survivors' group in Washington. Now, I plan to make working with this population my career.

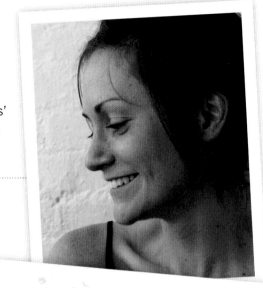

Dan Miller

Silverthorne, Colorado

I live by living. I love by loving. And I am courageous courageously. That was Julie's philosophy in dealing with cancer. I took this photo in 2006, five years after Julie's breast cancer had progressed to stage IV, and 18 years after her initial diagnosis. To me, the light in her eyes reflects the peace and joy she found by accepting her mortality. By "accepting mortality," I don't mean that she had lost the will to live—quite the opposite! For her, this acceptance was key to living fearlessly and fully in the present.

As Tolkien put it, "All we have to decide is what to do with the time that is given us." Through Julie's cancer, we learned gratitude and compassion. We learned to let go of being right, to find solace in nature, and to find comfort in open, heartfelt communication. Thanks, Julie!

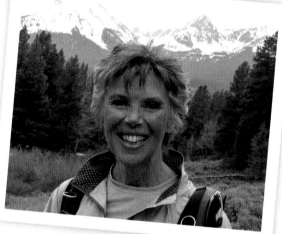

Live By Living offers outdoor activities (such as hiking, snowshoeing, survivor retreats) in the Colorado Rockies for cancer survivors and their caregivers.

Donna Hughes

Rockland County, New York

Sure, there is always an ache, pain, or worry, but every day alive just gets better and better!

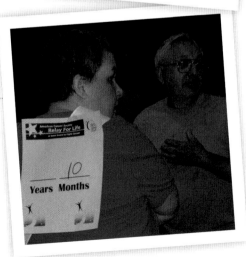

Jillian McDonald

New York, New York

I had bone cancer when I was 14 living in Canada, and I fought it with surgery, radiation, and chemotherapy. Since then, I finished high school, went to college, moved to New York City, pursued a master's degree, became an artist, and began teaching at a college. I am lucky enough to love what I do. Last year, I got tenure. This year, I am on sabbatical, traveling and researching. I make artwork that is fun and collaborative, and I meet the most wonderful people.

Every year I forget a little more about my former life as a cancer patient, but each October, I celebrate with someone special. I run to raise money for cancer research, have a party, go camping, or have a beautiful dinner. I don't know if life would be different without cancer, but I feel lucky every day.

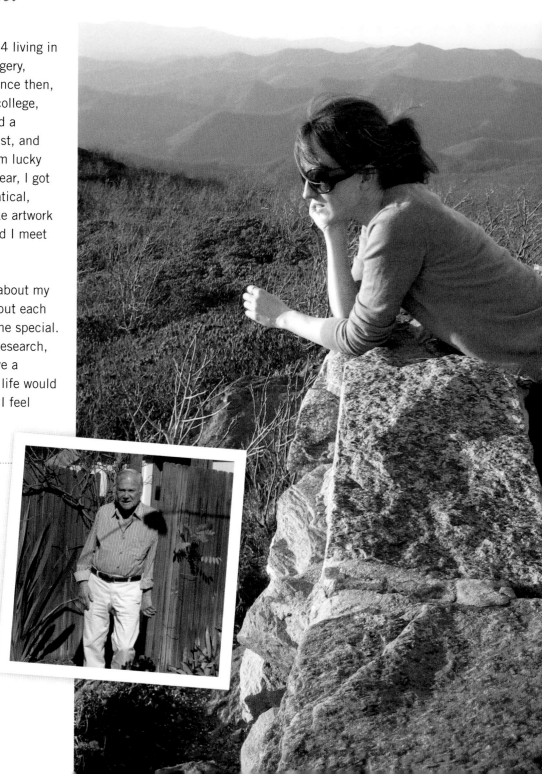

Gerald Schwartz

New York, New York

Better than ever. Everything moves at a more enjoyable pace for me.

Karen Siegel

Michigan

Fifteen years after my first cancer diagnosis, I thought I was done. I avoided radiation, which would have put me at higher risk for breast cancer. I gave birth to a beautiful girl, and I have treasured each moment with her. I thought of myself as a person, not a survivor.

Then, 19 years later, I was diagnosed with breast cancer.

I will always feel like a cancer survivor. My focus on a healthy diet and exercise is stronger. I will never again forget to maintain a good balance between work, home, and rest. I've found a tremendous amount of relief from complementary therapies. The support from my friends and family is humbling.

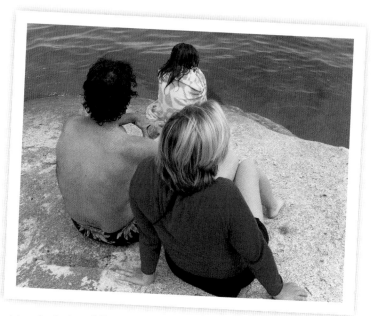

Wendy Harpham

United States

I was a busy doctor with three young children when I was diagnosed with lymphoma in 1990. I've been in and out of treatment ever since. Cancer has helped me know both the fragility and the hopes of life, and with that knowledge I live most fully.

This photo was taken in 1993, the day before leaving to participate in a clinical trial. Then, my life expectancy was about two years. Now, 17 years later, my cancer is in remission. I'm planning the weddings of my two daughters, a joy I didn't expect to experience when I entered the trial.

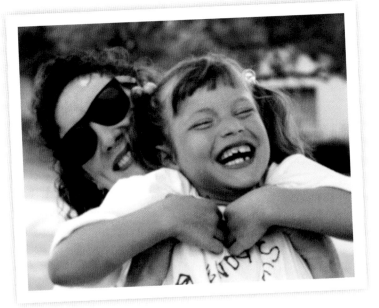

I devote my days to writing and speaking to patients and professionals about how patients can become healthy survivors, by which I mean people who receive good care and live as fully as possible. My life may be nothing like I expected or planned, and yet, life is good.

Will Cronenwett

Chicago, Illinois

Help. This is all moving so fast. I was diagnosed with cancer just three weeks ago. Now, one surgery and many appointments later, doctors are telling me that my chances are good. I haven't even gotten used to the word yet, and already, I might be a survivor? This feels like it's happening to somebody else. I don't know what to feel, and I don't know whom I can talk to about it.

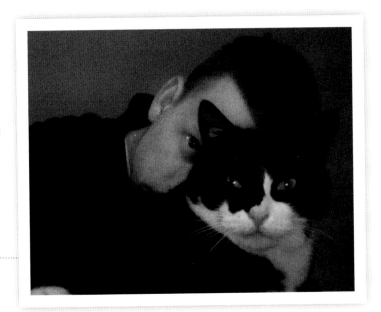

Nancy Blumenthaler

Akron, Ohio

My stage IV breast cancer diagnosis was terrifying because I have always taken care to make healthy choices. I have surrounded myself with good friends and family, and I am fighting, fighting, fighting every step of the way. Now, I understand there is no way to perfectly guard against illness or disease, but there is a way to live well, no matter what!

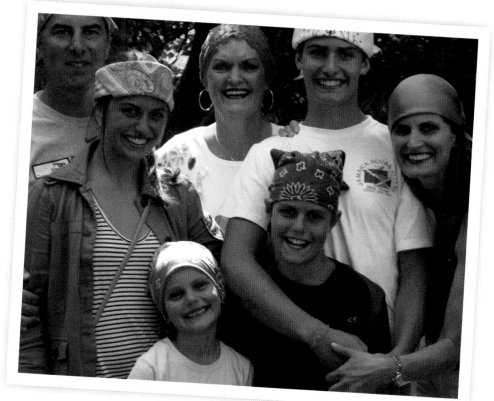

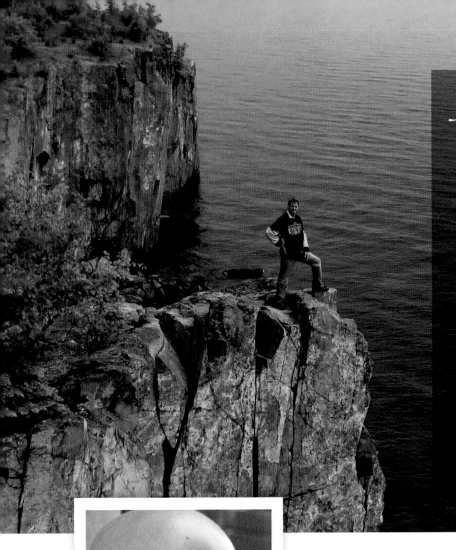

Ken Hirte

Lake Superior, Minnesota

I no longer *have* to do anything. I get to do everything, such as walk, eat fruits and vegetables, and live a good, healthy life. I am the luckiest person in the world. Six weeks after the removal of a fist-sized, stage III renal cell carcinoma, I was hiking several miles a day. I am healthier than ever.

This new lease on life provides me with perspective to truly appreciate those who love and care about me. A brush with mortality makes everything clear. I crave more time with energy-giving people, and I am trying to find ways to spend less time with energy-draining people and petty matters.

Adrienne Rathert

New Orleans, Louisiana

Six months after I finished cancer treatment, I accomplished two physical feats that I never imagined I would do. I hiked down and back up the Grand Canyon in one day, and a week later, I completed my first half marathon. Going through a year of chemotherapy with a smile gave me the strength to know I could get through anything with grace. I am currently working toward my master's degree in public health so that I can work with others in compromised health situations.

SARAH LEWERT

Keren Batiyov

Arlington, Virginia

I was diagnosed with breast cancer in October 2007 and had a bilateral mastectomy two months later. Ten days after my surgery, on December 25th, I was getting ready to go out for a "Jewish Christmas" (Chinese food and a movie) with friends. I was putting on my makeup and, suddenly, I became transfixed with my image in the mirror—my a-ha moment. It was the first time in my life that I really liked the person and the body that was reflected back at me.

I jokingly say that if all it took were the removal of a couple of appendages to like myself and my body, I'd have had the mastectomy years earlier. That's what's different—I like who I am, and I like my body. Who would have imagined?

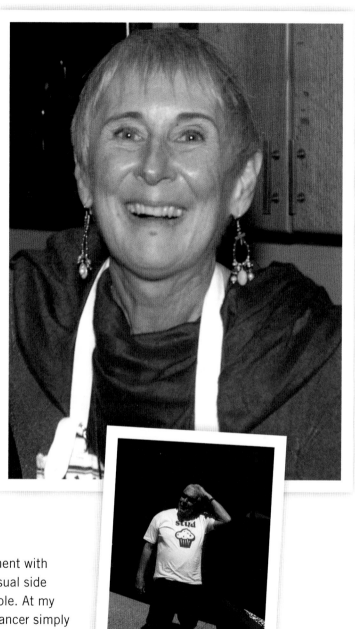

Dick Givens

Menlo Park, California

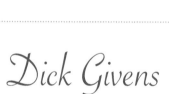

I have advanced prostate cancer. Treatment with radiation and medication has had the usual side effects; they are annoying but manageable. At my age, mortality questions are common. Cancer simply helps clarify the questions and the answers. The things I worried about most before cancer were really not as important as I had once thought—not to say they were shallow, but rather they really didn't matter. What does matter? To me, it's family.

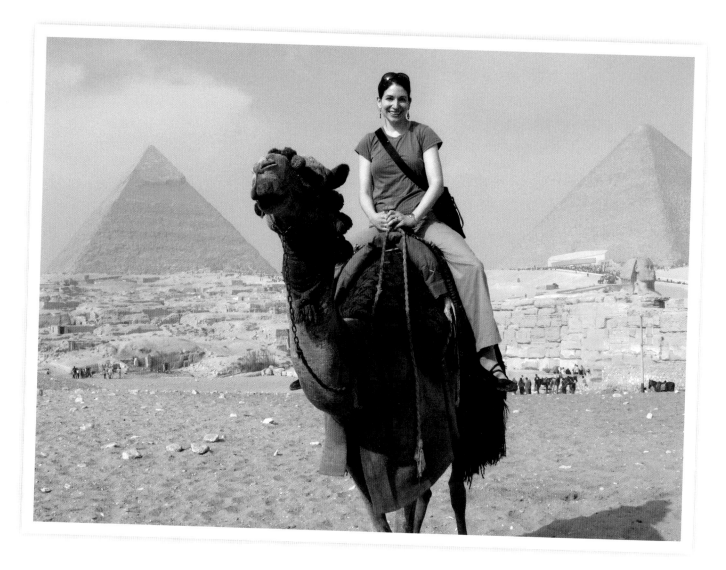

Allison Aab

Cairo, Egypt

Scars may heal, blood counts may normalize, years may pass. But never again will the simple act of waking up to a normal, boring day as a healthy individual be taken for granted, nor go unappreciated.

Carol Radsprecher

Brooklyn, New York

Diagnosed with stage I breast cancer 11 years ago (and counting), I am forever thankful to the staff at Memorial Sloan-Kettering Cancer Center for the treatment I received there.

While cancer is never far from my mind, I am appreciative of my mate, my friends, and my being able to make and show my paintings, drawings, and Photoshop work. I value life more than ever before.

I'd much prefer to have never had cancer, and I am not one to say it was a blessing in disguise. But having had it—and with the hope that I'll never "taste" that experience again—I am perhaps a little more appreciative of being alive than if I had never been through this. I am, for sure, more empathetic toward other people with cancer.

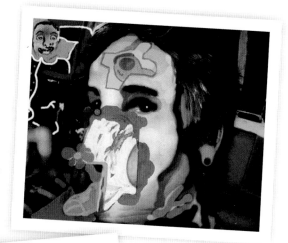

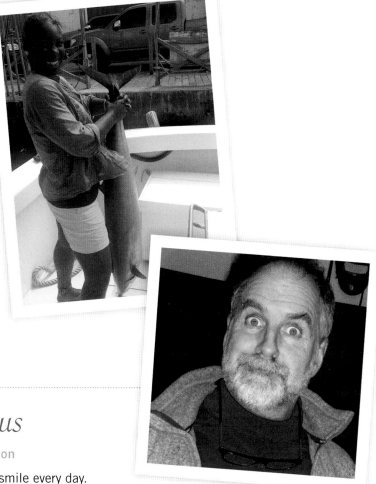

Ashley Jobe

Elon, North Carolina

I play rugby, *hard*. I serve as the opinions editor for my college newspaper, *The Pendulum*. I am a proud Make-A-Wish kid. I dance with zeal, laugh until I can't anymore, and step outside to breathe and remind myself I'm alive. I have a passion for travel, for food, and for love. My faith is stronger than ever, and I will never stop thanking God for the one invaluable gift I have been given—my family!

I kicked angiosarcoma's butt!

John Backus

Seattle, Washington

I celebrate with a smile every day.

Karen Farley

New York

This is a photo of my wonderful family!

When I was pregnant with my lovely daughter, Dana, I had end-stage lymphoma in my organs and bone marrow. I used a combination of conventional medicine and complementary therapies to help me get well. And that was 19 years ago!

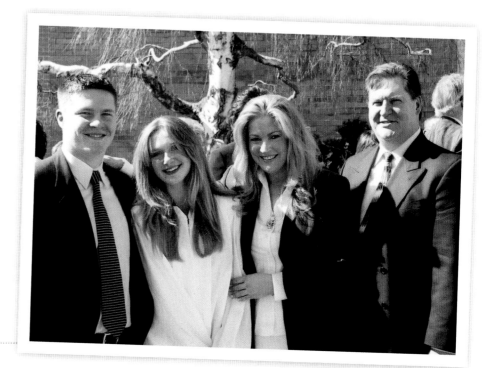

Mary Beth Miller

Little Compton, Rhode Island

I am managing to live with my very rare cancer. I may never technically be in the "survivor" category; I honestly don't like that word.

Cancer has changed my life for the better! My sweetie and I got married last month. We cherish our friends and family, and we find beauty in each and every moment. I can say that I'm surviving cancer's "inconveniences" by living my life to the fullest possible extent!

Mary Beth Miller was a registered horticultural therapist and founder of Gardening for Good. It was her mission to connect people to nature and provide "garden therapy." She often referred to her own garden as her piece of paradise on Earth. On August 8, 2010, Mary Beth left her earthly paradise for her heavenly paradise.

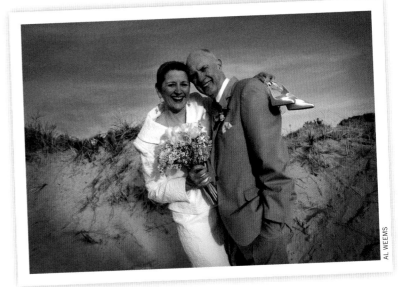

AL WEEMS

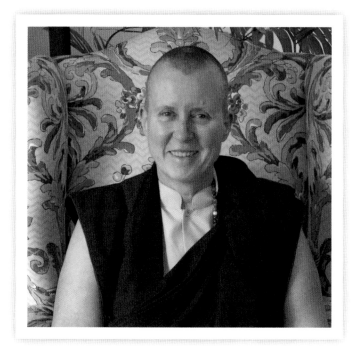

Khenmo Drolma

Vermont

Cancer was a gift of courage. I left my traditional life and became a Buddhist nun. I spent time in India and met the greatest spiritual masters of our time.

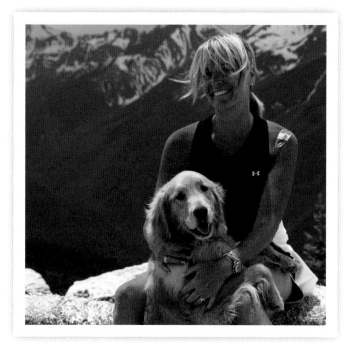

Robin Benjamin

Chatham, New Jersey

I have Waldenström macroglobulinemia, a form of non-Hodgkin lymphoma. It's a kind of lymphoma that is treatable but not curable. For me, there is no life *after* cancer. I've learned to live *with* it. And I understand that we all have something; we just don't know it yet.

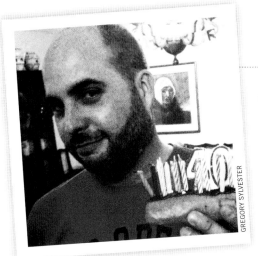

GREGORY SYLVESTER

Michael Pepper

New York, New York

I am more aware of what is important, and I keep those people and things close to me. Life is precious, and it is meant to be enjoyed!

Roxann Zarchin

California

I had stage IIA invasive lobular breast cancer. I am still shocked, as I never felt it. I am thankful it was found during a routine mammogram.

Now, I look at the world through grateful eyes. I try to get out more and enjoy nature. I take that strenuous hike I might not have tried before. Before cancer, I might have said, "Oh, I can't do that," but now I feel like I *must* do that!

I miss my hair; it seems to be taking a long time to return. In the big picture, the loss of my hair seems like a small price to pay.

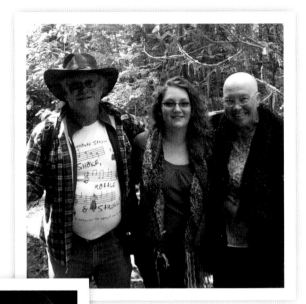

Ruud Van Soest

Chicago, Illinois

I had Hodgkin disease and was successfully treated with chemotherapy, radiation, and a splenectomy.

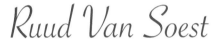

The nicest feeling I have after this experience is my appreciation of nature! I really have tremendous fun feeling the seasons change, seeing and hearing the birds and leaves, and smelling flowers. It's such a nice feeling!

Tim Dye

Syracuse, New York

Eight years cancer free.

Life's too short to stand still. Do something good in the world: help people in developing countries who have cancer. They have few options facing the disease. I've been to more than 20 countries and 5 continents since my cancer diagnosis.

There's much to do in the short lives we have.

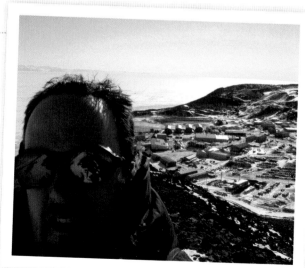

Lori J. Gowdy

Charlotte, North Carolina

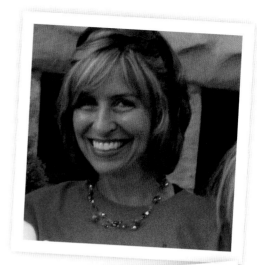

I love getting older. I love having hair. I love the taste of water.

Some people have asked if I was angry with God or felt it was unfair.
I tell them I felt gratitude. I was one of the lucky ones. I had a sister
and close friends who were there to hold my hand if I needed it.

I look back at my time living with cancer and think of it as a blessing.
Sure, there are things I lost, but I gained more, including the realization
that I am mortal. Life is short and although there are rough moments,
I need not be anxious. God provides what I need. I am eating more
fruits and vegetables. I celebrate with wine more often. I enjoy the
children I spend my days with as a teacher. Each day is a gift!

Lucy G. Lehman

Chicago, Illinois

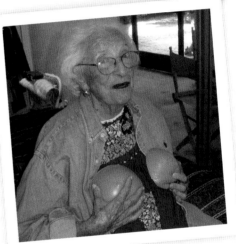

My mother, Edith Ganford, had a mastectomy at age 75. She died (not
of cancer) this past January at the age of 99. She was lucky because
she was able to live her life as fully as her age would allow, never losing
her sense of humor.

Jerry Joern

Afghanistan

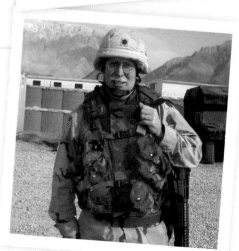

I was able to go on after my serious fight with cancer and serve my
country—both in Afghanistan and in New Orleans, Louisiana, after
Hurricane Katrina. Having a new lease on life helps me focus on
the ones I care about and allows me to help other people with
a grateful spirit.

Denise Silverstone

Nicaragua

I have been struggling to understand how life is different for me after cancer. I thought there was going to be one definitive emotion. But now I know, as with most things in life, there are layers and complexities and a healthy balance of good and bad.

On the good side, I know what it means to be truly grateful for supportive friends and family. And I have also learned a great deal about accepting what life gives you and finding a way to get through it.

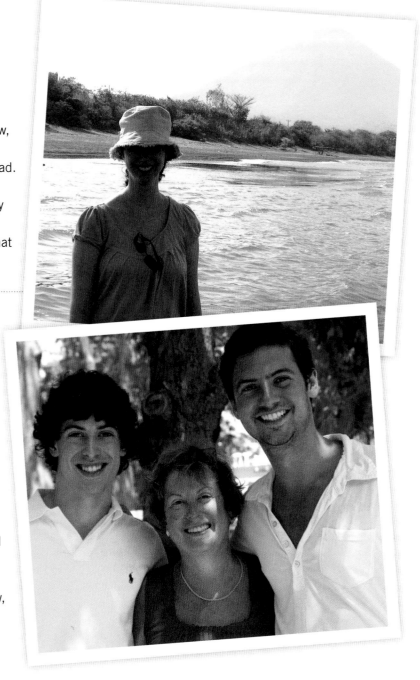

Jane C. Bressler

New York, New York

I had breast cancer in 2000. I had a mastectomy, reconstruction, and chemotherapy. Then, I saw three doctors every six months and was fine. In 2001, my husband died of metastatic bladder cancer.

I thought I was a "survivor" until December 2008, when I was diagnosed with metastatic breast cancer in my liver and bones. It was a total shock to everyone. Now, I am living with breast cancer. I have treatments weekly, and I am treasuring every minute I feel well, which, for now, is most of the time.

I spend as much time as possible with my wonderful sons seen in this picture, my two grandsons, and my newborn granddaughter. I do the things I really want to do, especially travel—my next trip is to Africa.

But I do still wonder what will happen when this and then other treatments fail.

Joan Morrissey

Ontario, Canada

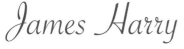

I discovered the sport of dragon boating. I'm part of a breast cancer survivor team. It makes me feel strong because I had to conquer my fear of water to participate. I value my friends and say yes to every opportunity to participate in social activities. I'm traveling to all the places I want to visit. My work/life balance is much healthier now.

James Harry

Salt Lake City, Utah

I am so much more aware of my mortality!

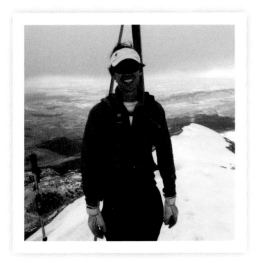

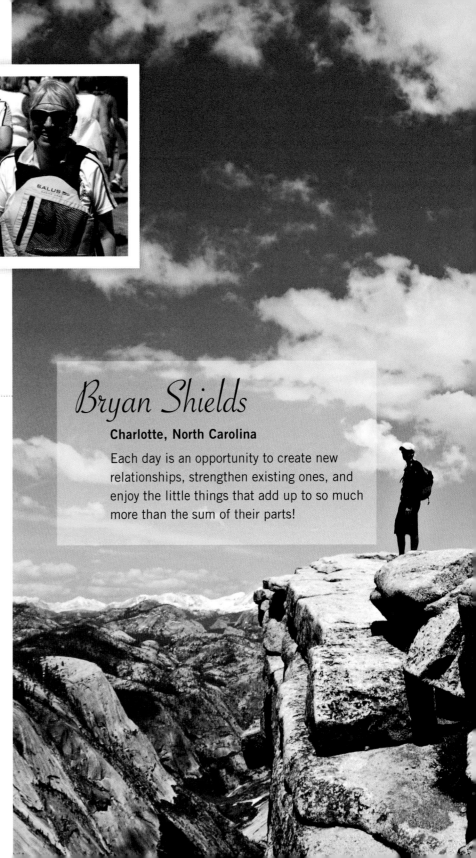

Bryan Shields

Charlotte, North Carolina

Each day is an opportunity to create new relationships, strengthen existing ones, and enjoy the little things that add up to so much more than the sum of their parts!

Sandra Elliott

Claremont, California

Life is painful. I now have problems doing simple things like walking and standing—things I once took for granted. I have more compassion for people who are limited physically. I now know firsthand what suffering means. I get joy from the smallest things now. Every day.

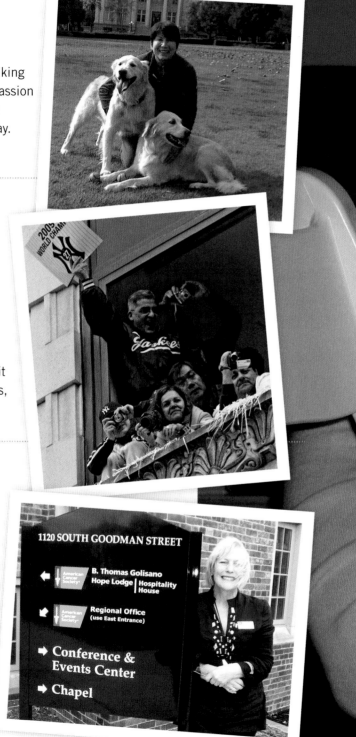

Steve Scalici

New York, New York

Is my life different? Completely. But the process of understanding just to what degree it is different was a slow one. Before, I was fussy, isolated, standoffish, a perfectionist, and sometimes sullen. After cancer, I requested help when I needed it. I was funny, gregarious, and less serious. And my photo says it all—celebratory—not just for the 2009 World Champion Yankees, but also for life!

Lorraine Clements

Rochester, New York

Who would have thought that breast cancer treatment would lead me to the best job of my life? Attending a Look Good...Feel Better® program provided by the American Cancer Society led me to eventually become the director of the Hope Lodge® Hospitality House. Hope Lodge provides free lodging for cancer patients who travel for their cancer treatments. It's an opportunity for me to give back and provide hope that so many people need when they travel the road of cancer. I feel so fortunate to be able to share my journey and provide encouragement to all who walk that common road.

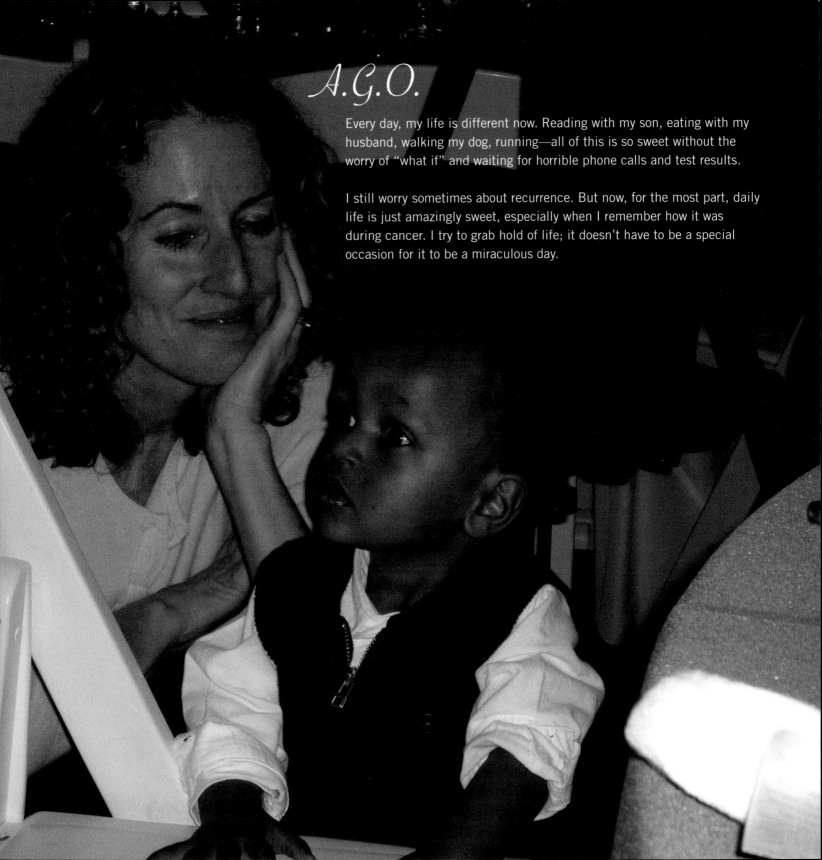

A.G.O.

Every day, my life is different now. Reading with my son, eating with my husband, walking my dog, running—all of this is so sweet without the worry of "what if" and waiting for horrible phone calls and test results.

I still worry sometimes about recurrence. But now, for the most part, daily life is just amazingly sweet, especially when I remember how it was during cancer. I try to grab hold of life; it doesn't have to be a special occasion for it to be a miraculous day.

John Brockman

Cincinnati, Ohio

At age 59, I have been in remission for five years from non-Hodgkin lymphoma. I can say that I am extremely lucky, but I realize my luck is not that I had cancer. It's that I survived without negative side effects. I have a loving wife, family, friends, and coworkers whom I love and who love me. I had all this before I had cancer, but surviving cancer has made me appreciate it so much more.

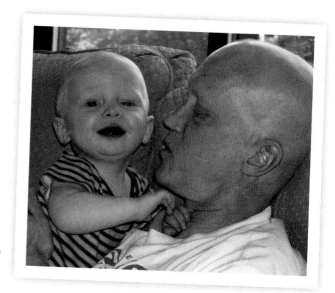

I am in remission now, but this particular cancer tends to come back. Every six months, I go get scanned and then wait to see if it has come back. My hope is that I survive long enough to see my grandson graduate from college. So far, so good.

Karissa Schecter

Charlotte, North Carolina

I find that the experience of having had cancer colors every aspect of my life. I am plagued by a fear of recurrence that recedes at times, only to surge to the surface once again. I try to keep it at bay by reminding myself that there is little I can do to affect my future other than to live healthily and be vigilant. I try to remain in the present.

At the same time, I have learned that I am stronger than I thought, and I can do things that I never thought myself capable of. I no longer take my health for granted, and I try my best to keep my family healthy as well. Life is so precious to me; I am holding on as tightly as I can.

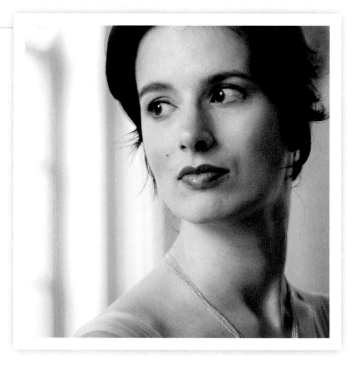

Elizabeth Susan Hooper

Corvallis, Oregon

My body has been altered, and I have chronic pain. However, it doesn't stop me from enjoying the simple moments, such as hearing the hundreds of frogs croaking in our back field or the taste of my morning coffee while I chat with friends on Facebook. Most important, I don't take for granted the love my family has for me because I know, no matter what, it is eternal.

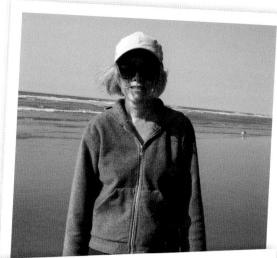

Evelyn LaRoche

Rhode Island

I appreciate and love my family more. I try to enjoy life and live one day at a time. With God's help, I hope I continue to live the rest of my life in good health.

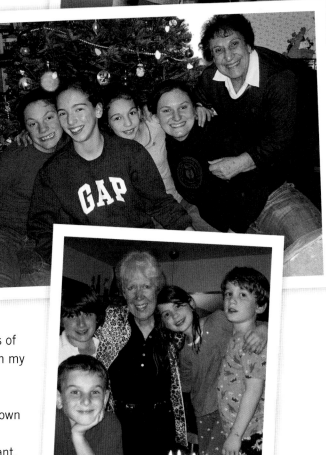

Diane Levinson

San Carlos, California

For me, the new century began with two separate episodes of breast cancer. In the meantime, I lost my parents and then my younger brother to pancreatic cancer.

Here I am, 10 years later, with seven little people (four shown in this picture) that keep me going—my West Coast grandchildren. They keep me young despite a breast implant, eye lens implants, and hip replacements. In sunny Northern California, I am bionic and going strong!

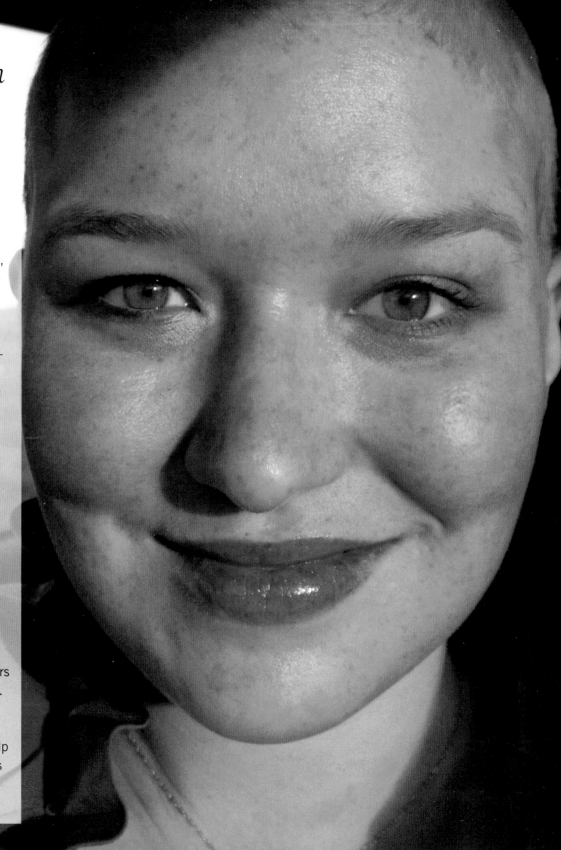

Ruth Buchanan

Portland, Oregon

After two rounds with non-Hodgkin lymphoma and a stem cell transplant, I am wry and a little bit unsettled. Being on the brink of death and constantly reminded of my meager chances of survival, all I can tolerate is passion and nothing less.

There is no room in my life—no matter its length—for apathy, reluctance, or entitlement. I have lost the capacity to understand or tolerate these attitudes in others.

I was diagnosed after graduating from an expensive college in the midst of a collapsed job market, and now all I can stomach is an impactful, engaged, and interesting career with a nonprofit organization.

After cancer, all that matters is what and whom you love. I married my partner, and we're taking off to travel, love, and live. I hope to help eradicate the stigma of this disease and improve my community somehow.

Kaethe Weingarten

Boston, Massachusetts

I jumped off a 35-foot cliff to show that cancer makes every day difficult. I have survived three cancers in 21 years. My motto? Turn private pain into public purpose.

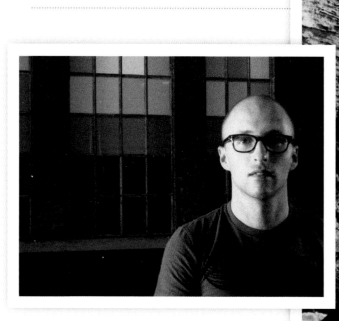

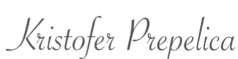

Kristofer Prepelica

Jersey City, New Jersey

Like many survivors, I am more comfortable with my own mortality, but there are also flashes of anxiety regarding recurrence. This is the unspoken legacy of survival that is difficult to explain to those who never went through cancer diagnosis and treatment.

Paulette Carles

Petaluma, California

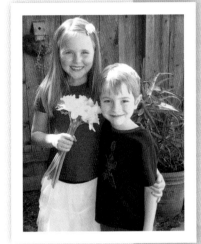

Isabel is a strong, smart, lovely child. You would never be able to pick her out of a lineup as the kid who fought cancer. Isabel has a younger brother, Gabriel, who bore witness to the countless tears, worry, and terror we experienced throughout the roller coaster of his sister's harsh chemotherapy treatments.

Isabel and Gabriel are the best of friends, and their bond has only been strengthened by this ordeal. After two and a half years of constant chemotherapy, Isabel is now a happy, healthy 8-year-old who loves the third grade, drawing, and reading. At such young ages, these children know what truly matters in life. As a family, we don't sweat the small stuff. We're poor as dirt, but happy as can be because we know all that matters is health, happiness, and family. These two children will make a difference in this world and are already giving back.

Sandy Scott

Seminole, Florida

I extract the most I can out of each and every day. I have an extra keen appreciation for life and my incredible health and athleticism.

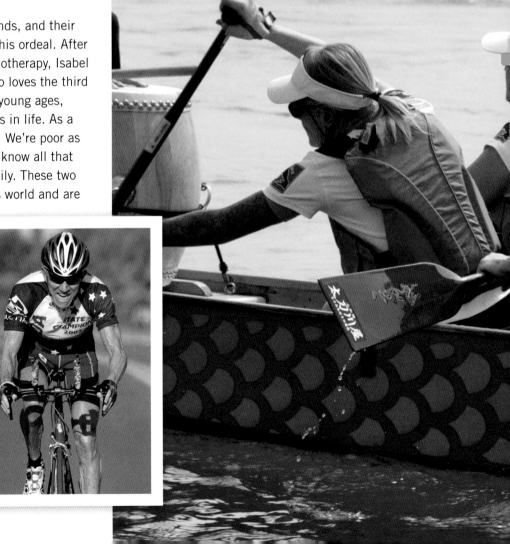

Lenore Spelbring

California

After finishing treatment, I joined a group of women cancer survivors who race dragon boats. Now, my focus is on wellness and being grateful for the extra time I have been given.

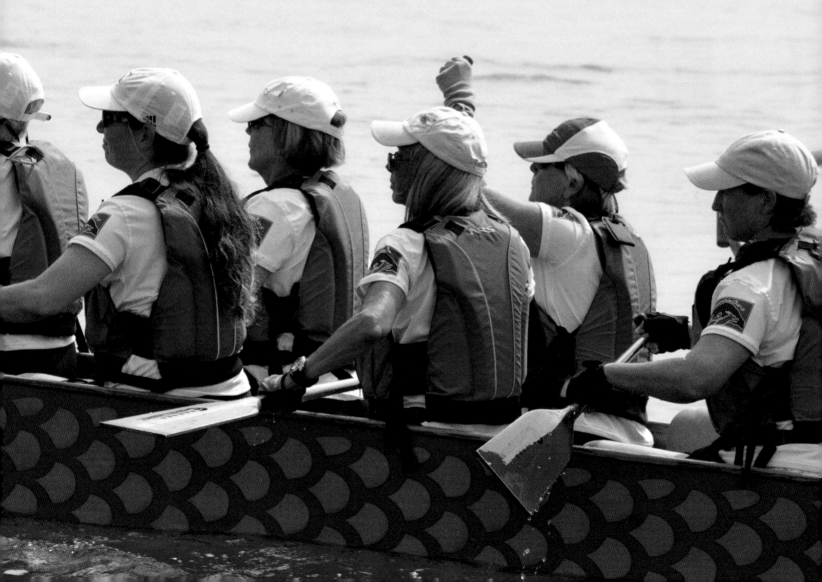

Shruti Modi

Pennsylvania

I am a three-year survivor. I love life and my time with my kids, husband, family, and friends. I keep a good work–life balance. I still can't believe that God gave me a second chance to live! I appreciate my life the second time around.

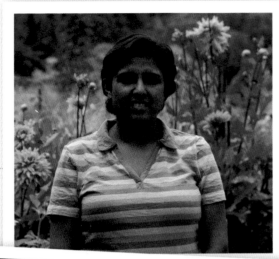

Kairol Rosenthal

Chicago, Illinois

During treatment, I created my "drama-reduction program." Cancer was a major crisis over which I often had no control. And I desperately wanted to squelch any extra ounce of calamity that I could.

I dissolved relationships with high-maintenance friends and acquaintances. I felt guilty and selfish at first, but the more I did it, the easier it became. The results were phenomenal. As my physical and mental world spiraled out of control, I downsized my work and social life to an even-keeled platform of support.

Now, instead of the charismatic, melodramatic guys I used to date, I'm married to a stable and caring man whom I adore. Instead of dealing with prima donna coworkers, I love my new, solitary profession writing about young adult cancer. Living with this disease has taught me that when it comes to the flamboyancy of life, sometimes less is more.

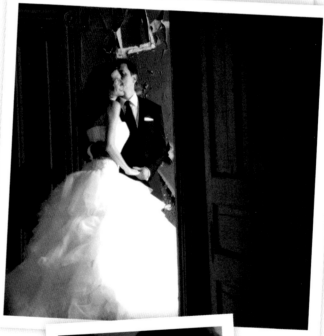

Ian Hoggard

San Antonio, Texas

I am able to play with my baby brother, Chad (on the right). I can go to school. I am able to go on vacations with my family. I can be a kid again.

Susan Muniak

Napa, California

I had stage III, grade 3 endometrial cancer, followed by a complete hysterectomy, chemotherapy, and radiation. I also had lymphedema, weekly scraping, diarrhea, neuropathy, radiation proctitis, weight gain, and saw my "rock" say goodbye.

In some ways, I wouldn't trade going through cancer for anything. I work more creatively. I relish my time with family and friends. I see more clearly. I challenge myself every day. It is good to be alive. The ultimate lesson? Embrace it, because it's your cancer; it has a lot to teach you.

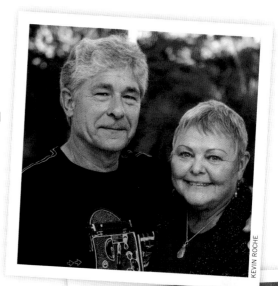

KEVIN ROCHE

Nancy Crane

Hinsdale, Massachusetts

I just hit my five-year mark. Cancer helped me figure out what was really important to me.

Veronica Foster

Wilton, Connecticut

I still swim half a mile, four days a week during the summer. I ski three days a week in the winter, and I walk for two hours, four days a week in the spring and fall. The only difference, now, is that the intensity with which I write has mellowed.

I tell friends that there were only 12 drops of blood on six different days that indicated I had uterine cancer. This symptom ceased long before my positive biopsy. So, I remind friends to pay attention to details.

My grandson's birth and his aunt's wedding made the summer of 2009, when I had my surgery, a joyous one.

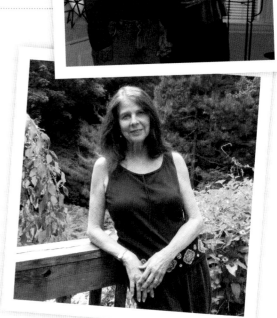

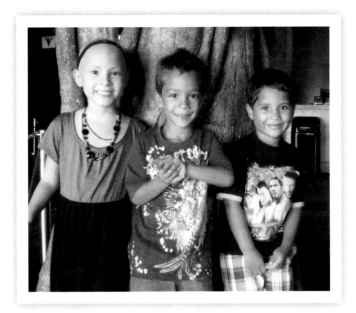

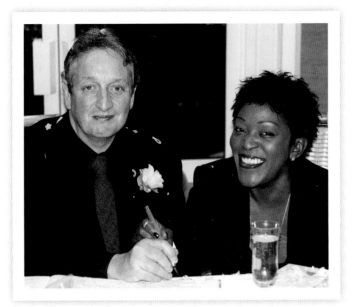

Brenda L. Molina

Caguas, Puerto Rico

After her diagnosis of acute myeloid leukemia in May 2010 and the intense treatment that followed, Livangeli Barreto-Molina showed our family that she is blessed by God. In her worst moments, she managed to keep her smile and happiness. She is now undergoing her last consolidation treatment and is doing great. Cancer changed her and our family forever, but we are stronger now, faithful people, and we want to help others in the same situation.

Anthony Firmin

Manchester, England

This is me and my wife on our wedding day. She passed away exactly three months later after battling breast cancer for eight years. I miss her desperately. She was my soulmate and my best friend.

I was diagnosed with bowel and liver cancer five years ago. Now, I am studying for a photography degree.

Doris Taylor

Sacramento, California

I have never been so busy! I volunteer five days a week, and I am very active. My daughter, mom, sister, brother, and nephew have all died of lung cancer. So, I am one of the lucky ones!

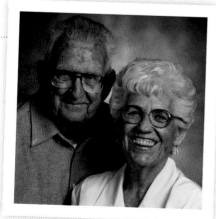

Helen Palmquist

Lincolnshire, Illinois

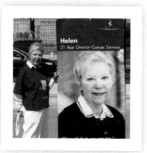

I was diagnosed with stage IIIC ovarian cancer in 1987 when I was 41. I had two major surgeries and two and a half years of chemotherapy. I had a recurrence in 1993, but I have not needed treatment since March of 1994.

My mission is to give hope to those going through this experience. I needed hope, and I tell others, "If I did it, you can, too." I have made wonderful friends among my ovarian "sisters." By giving, I have received so much in return.

Lily Mulcahy

Boston, Massachusetts

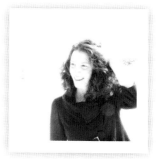

When I was 18, I was diagnosed with thyroid cancer. When I was 19, the doctors found it had metastasized, and they told me I would live with it for the rest of my life. Even though my prognosis was very good, it took a long time for me to feel safe again.

Cancer brought me a sense of wonder I don't think I would ever have experienced otherwise. My family is more precious to me than I ever imagined, and now I realize my importance to them. Best of all, I feel purposeful, safe, and surrounded by beauty. Of course, that's just how I feel today. Luckily, nothing else matters.

Barbara Kallaur

Indiana

I celebrated the first anniversary of my cancer surgery by playing a concert with a wonderful friend for a lovely audience. A year before, I had no idea whether this would even be possible.

Like many professional classical musicians, I have been plagued by perfectionist "bullies." That has changed; now, it is just a joy to play. As I write, I see fledglings in the nest outside my kitchen window, and the irises and coral bells are in bloom. Life is sweet.

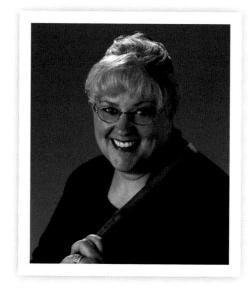

Brechin Flournoy

California

Breast cancer grounded me in the immediacy of life and the joy that it offers. Every day, the mirror reminds me that I am a part of this world—that my mother's story is not my own.

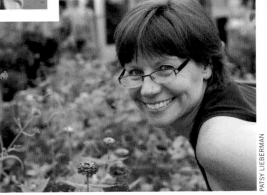

Christine Rathbun

United States

Vivid, finite, fierce.
Angry, hungry, annealed.
Precarious.
Grand.
Sweet.
Blessed.

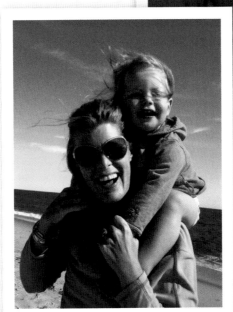

Beth Py-Lieberman

Silver Spring, Maryland

Cancer is just another way of saying, "Life is short." I waste not a single moment now. Life is so sweet, so good, and so fleeting.

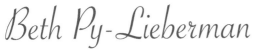

PATSY LIEBERMAN

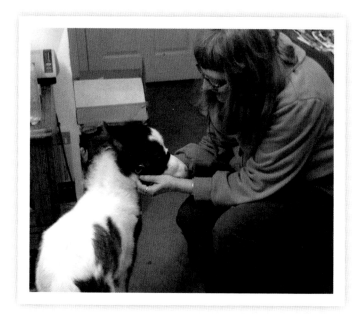

Victoria Brownlee

West Virginia

It's like I see with new eyes and hear with new ears, even though I do miss the things I can no longer do. I am a 15-year breast cancer survivor and a 12-year survivor of cervical cancer.

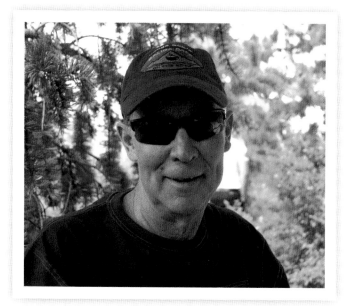

Thomas H. Haberthier

Colorado

My days are fuller and felt more deeply now. Instead of it being just another day, I now feel time passing by.

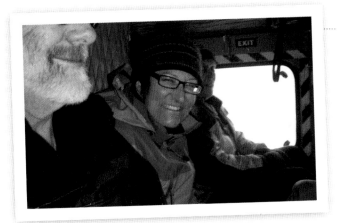

Karen Ruterford

British Columbia, Canada

I'm bolder, braver, and louder! Life is worth living. I see things I never took the time to notice before. Colors seem brighter, more vivid. I appreciate the wonder of youth. I love life!

Angela Olsen

Raleigh, North Carolina

I never take moments for granted, whether it's rubbing my dog's belly, getting a call from my mom, holding hands with my husband, or riding in racecars with my 3-year-old son. Life is amazing. It is too short to be filled with stress or fear. I won't live forever, but I'm going to have fun while I'm here!

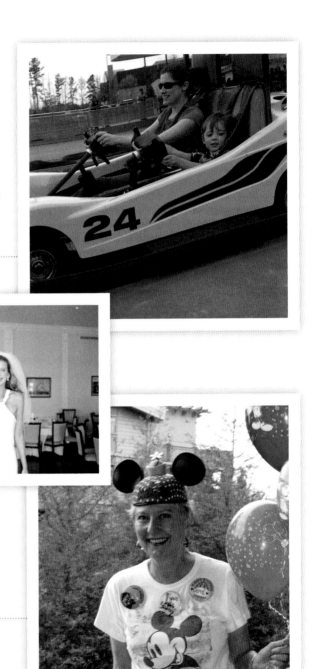

Edward Robert Alvarado

New York, New York

I was diagnosed with stage II vocal cord cancer on New Year's Eve of 2008. After three operations and five weeks of radiation, I recovered and regained the use of my voice.
Since I could not speak for weeks at a time during my treatment, I now appreciate every word I say. More important, before cancer, I always lamented the mistakes I made in my past. Now, I never think about them and truly realize the future is far more important!

Carol Wilder

Anaheim, California

I am much more able to delight in delight itself.

Cindy Elias

Auburn, Maine

Each day after cancer is a celebration. I have little patience for complaining. From the moment of my diagnosis, I received gifts of kindness, friendship, and laughter—gifts that cost nothing but were valued beyond measure. I give hugs to those who need them. I enjoy the sunrise and sunset, a crocus poking through the snow, the sun shining through the golden maple leaves of autumn and sparkling on a fresh winter snowfall. I am content to be with my family, to know that my children are happy, and to hold my first grandchild.

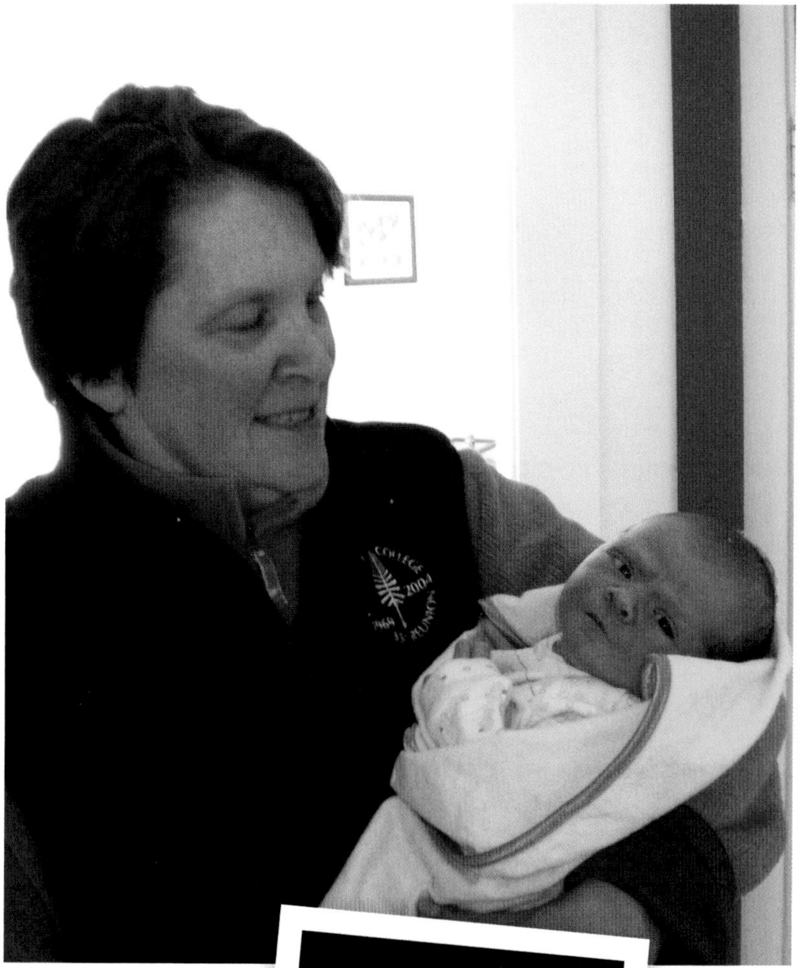

Amy Robins

San Diego, California

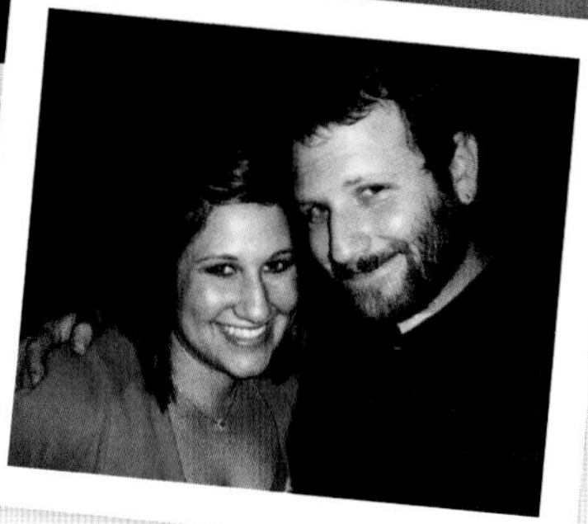

This sweet picture shows my two remaining children, the survivors. In my heart, I still have three kids. But Alex and Emily are still here while their brother, Sean, is not. Ewing sarcoma took him on November 17, 2006, at the age of 22. I can't really ever know how my survivors feel. The experience is different for a mother than for a sibling. But I wonder if they go to sleep or wake up thinking of him, as I do. I hope my Seany knows how much I miss him. But my precious survivors, Alex and Emily, they honor Sean every day with the work they do, the music they play, and the lives they live. I know, without a doubt, that Sean is proud of them. I love my survivors so much. I just wish Sean had been one of them, too.

Susan Schwalb

New York, New York

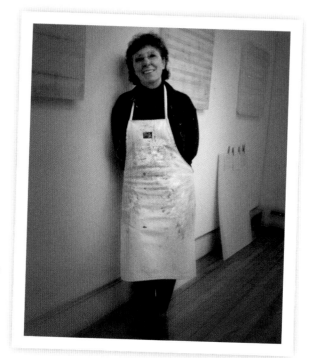

This photo is of me in my studio. I am an artist specializing in silverpoint paintings and drawings.

Since I had ductal carcinoma in situ and a mastectomy, I have been pedaling as fast as I can to make my artwork and continue my life as an artist. I am aware of how fragile life is and how important friends and family are. There are still dream trips I want to take, and I hope to take them.

I am part of an informal network of breast cancer patients. I help counsel friends (and there have been many) who join the breast cancer club. It is hard, since I relive my own cancer experience each time, but it is an important part of my life. If you have had cancer, there is always a chance of a recurrence, so I continue to cherish each day.

Harrie Bakst

New York, New York

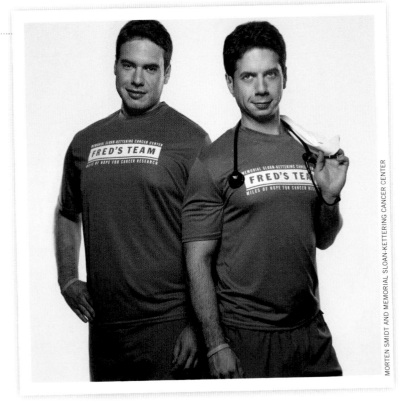

One side effect from my treatment was the loss of my taste buds. Everything tasted like cardboard, except for one thing—Coca-Cola.

After treatment ended (that's me on the left), my side effects diminished and my taste buds not only came back, but also came back enhanced. Every week since, I have a Coke to remind me just how good life is.

MORTEN SMIDT AND MEMORIAL SLOAN-KETTERING CANCER CENTER

Claire Chew

Venice, California

Twenty-four years after my last cancer treatment for Ewing sarcoma, my passion in life is helping clients transform loss and hardship into happiness. Cancer has taught me resiliency and empathy, strengths that propel me when I'm helping guide others through their pain. It is my belief that grief and loss are not only about death and dying, but also about every disappointment we have ever faced. I work with clients to heal the grief and loss of chronic illness, divorce, miscarriage, the loss of pets, or the deaths of loved ones.

Cancer has taught me to see life through a new lens. Cancer took away mobility in my right arm; now, I am ambidextrous. I didn't save my eggs at 19, and yet I overcame infertility challenges and became a mother at 40. Cancer has taught me to open my heart to the future with trust and optimism.

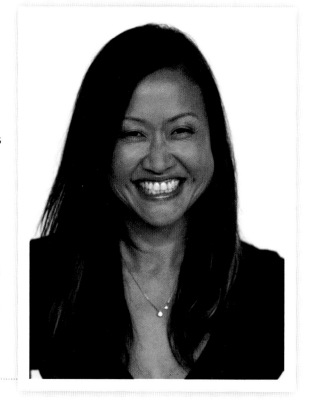

Karen Holmes

England

In April 2010, my daughter Hebe, age 14, was diagnosed with hepatocellular carcinoma. Before,

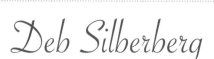

she was my stroppy teenage daughter, and now, she is the best friend I will ever have. Her strength and sense of humor give me the energy I need to face each day.

Deb Silberberg

New York, New York

I am grateful, but fearful that cancer may still shorten my life.

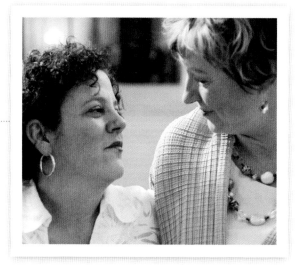

Joel Byersdorfer

Denver, Colorado

I have gained a greater appreciation of the ability to play. Endurance sports have always been important to me, and recovering from chemotherapy and a stem cell transplant has been a whole different type of race. I don't know what my "new" body is going to be capable of. The races are planned, the entry fees paid—so far, so good.

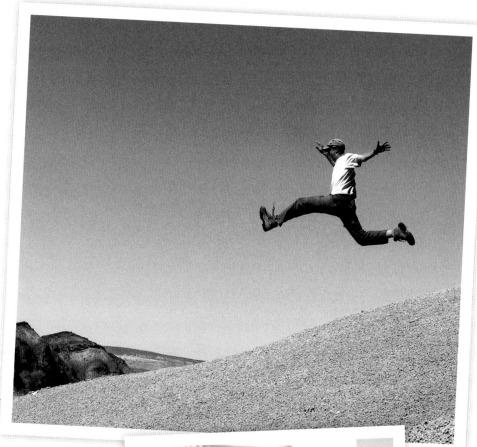

Doris Castro

Colombia

It's harder for me to be happy now. Though I haven't given up hope, cancer is always on my mind. Fear is always there, too—sadness and fear.

I know I am lucky that I'm cancer free now. However, I'm always sad and sometimes I don't even know why. I wish I could give uplifting messages to people in my situation, but what can I say? I keep fighting for myself to have joy and peace no matter what.

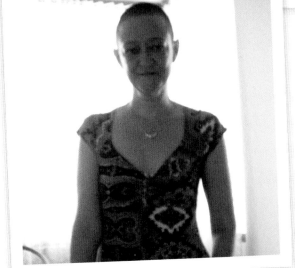

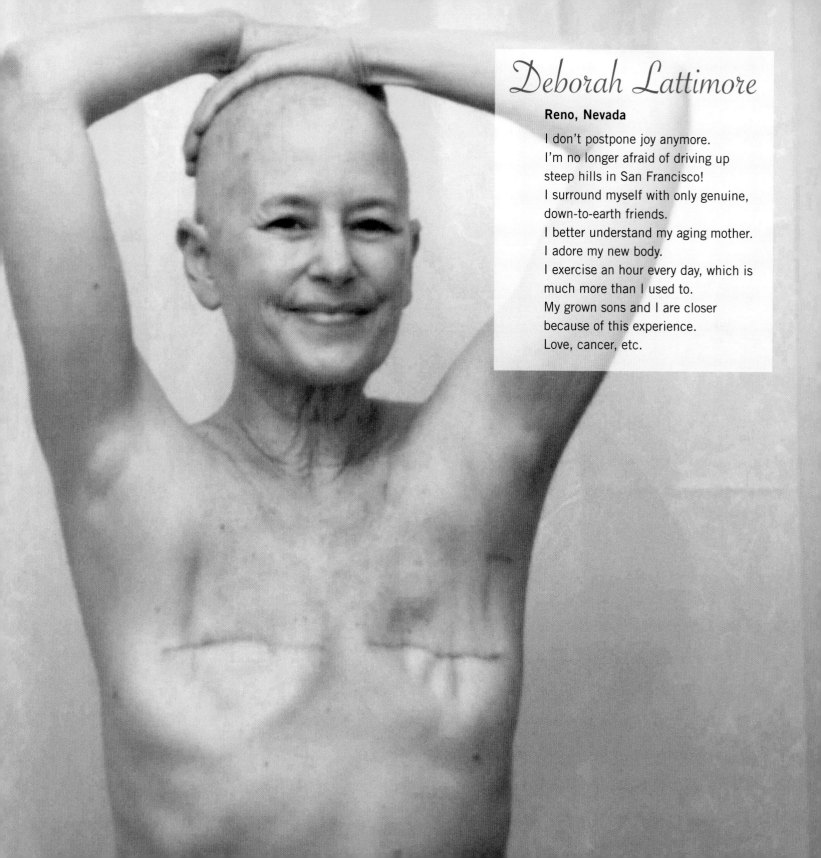

Deborah Lattimore

Reno, Nevada

I don't postpone joy anymore.
I'm no longer afraid of driving up
steep hills in San Francisco!
I surround myself with only genuine,
down-to-earth friends.
I better understand my aging mother.
I adore my new body.
I exercise an hour every day, which is
much more than I used to.
My grown sons and I are closer
because of this experience.
Love, cancer, etc.

Jeff Erdfarb

Teaneck, New Jersey

I have been in remission for six years after battling anal squamous cell carcinoma. I have had four good years, but the last two have been difficult because my immune system is breaking down because of the chemotherapy and radiation treatments. A day does not go by without some type of physical pain, but I am living life to the fullest. I treat every day as a new beginning and look forward to tomorrow's challenges. A great family and belief in God have helped, as well as my drive to succeed at my new business.

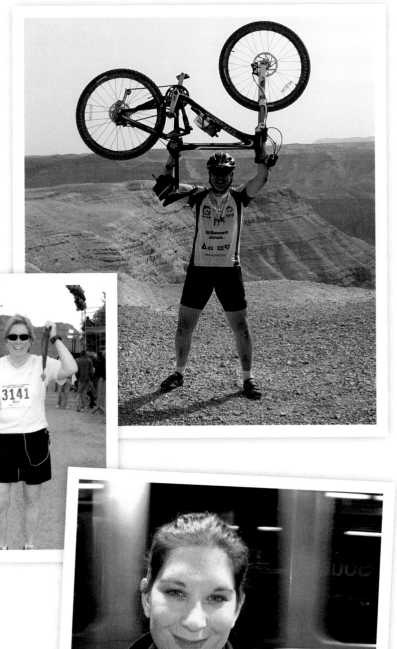

Shawn Williams

Lansing, Michigan

I'm no longer afraid of life. I've started running half marathons!

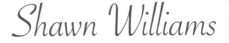

Ellen Miller

Chicago, Illinois

I can see what life is all about now.

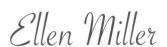

Maureen Shannon

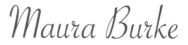

Ontario, Canada

My furry little friends understand living in the moment. There's no right or wrong in their world. There is just unconditional love for me—no matter where my thoughts are spinning off to or what is happening inside my body. They are my teachers.

Cancer has been living with me for 22 years, and I try to live in the moment each and every day. Life is a gift. Be kind.

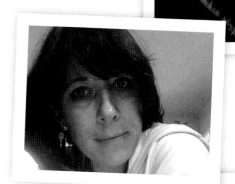

Maura Burke

California

It's still very new; it's only been three months since my surgery. The world feels upside down. Most days, I feel like I'm living in a kaleidoscope, and I'm looking out at the world from the inside. It's backward and jumbled. It's still beautiful, but I can't quite make sense of it yet.

Anna Drallios

Conodoguinet Creek, Pennsylvania

I had my last chemotherapy treatment for breast cancer this past July and am now considered cancer free.

When life becomes overwhelming and I'm harassed by daily aggravations, all I have to do is remember how it felt to live with cancer, and my heart leaps with joy that I am now cancer free.

Now, I have to strengthen myself spiritually and emotionally, so if the cancer comes back, it will not be so devastating.

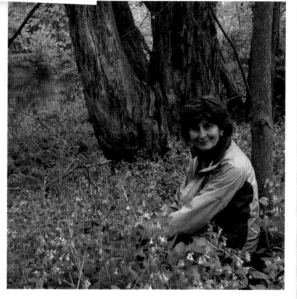

Heidi Rogers

Seattle, Washington

The gifts of cancer…

I cherish life.
I feel at ease with the thought of passing on.
The day-to-day idiosyncrasies I once took for granted are treasures.
I choose the people around me with purpose.
I am direct about all things and have grown to be tactful.
I laugh at my frustrations and mistakes.
I do what I love now, not tomorrow.
I found balance—in food, in life, in yoga, in school, in work.
I don't take anything too seriously.
I love more, more often and more deeply.

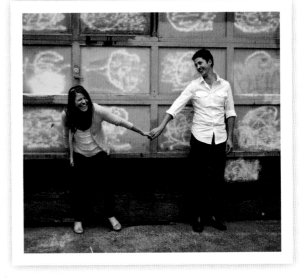

I have been in remission for 15 years. I wouldn't take back that scary experience of being a child with terminal cancer. It changed me and my closest friends and family to the core, and I believe for the better.

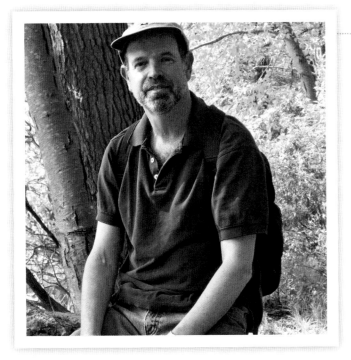

David Posner

New York, New York

I'm a physician, and I stepped onto the other side of the patient–doctor equation when I was diagnosed with cancer. I know now what it's like to be told you have cancer, what it's like to wait for the phone call with your latest CT scan results, what it's like to feel your heart sink. I'm a better physician—and person—for it.

I also learned how dinner with your wife and kids and coffee on a Sunday morning are all it takes to be in nirvana.

Laura McGinnis

Pittsburgh, Pennsylvania

The beginning of knowing comes in interpreting the first impression. We look upon others and begin the story.

My breast cancer diagnosis brought a shift in my self-perception. I looked even deeper inward as my outside began to fall apart. Others treated me differently.

I felt an urgency to pick up my camera. My comfort behind the lens changed, as I wanted my young sons to have a record of the time we spent together. With a photograph, we have the power to stop time. Looking into one, we can travel back to feel that moment.

I have a new identity as a survivor. I do not know what the future holds. My past has shaped me. Survivorship is a fight. Life is a gift. I got my first tattoo in celebration of completing treatment. Cancer has been my hidden dragon. The Chinese reads "dragon slayer."

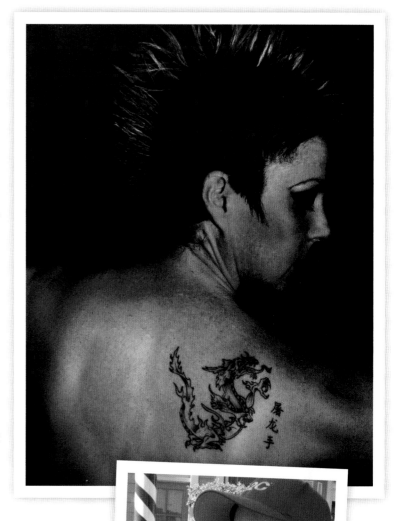

Jenn Michelle Pedini

Virginia

It's a little like being chased by a ghost. I'm always looking over my shoulder to see if cancer is lurking in the shadows. Some people live paycheck to paycheck; I think for many survivors, we live scan to scan.

Katherine Blossfield Iannitelli

Chicago, Illinois

When breast cancer made me face my mortality, I realized just how much I love and appreciate my family, my friends, and life itself. Fear and sadness made it difficult for me to get right back into the swing of things after cancer, but I know now that living in fear is not really living. Now, my daily mantra is to go out and live my life, imagine the best, and love the people around me every day!

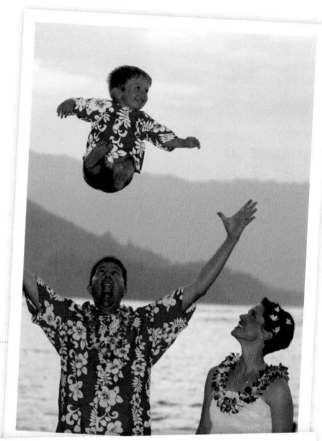

Jen Newlin

Oregon

In 36 days, it will have been a year. Ideally, there will be clear scans again. So, I'm simmering between "have" and "had" when it comes to cancer. And also between the tenses of love. But I am content in today. Celebrating the remarkable goodness in people, the onset of spring, and even that cup of glorious coffee. And slowly, I am learning to love again.

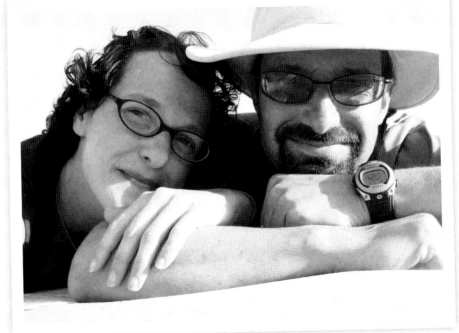

Jarratt Applewhite

New Mexico

My cancer was cured two years ago after I received a liver transplant. The cancer was caused by hepatitis C, which I have had for over 35 years. I am currently six months into my third attempt in the last 12 years to eliminate hepatitis from my body. It is too early to tell if the third time will be the charm.

Since I got a new liver, I've attended my youngest child's college graduation, welcomed two grandchildren into the world, and, next month, I will attend my oldest daughter's wedding. These extraordinary blessings frame my life and are a constant reminder of my good fortune.

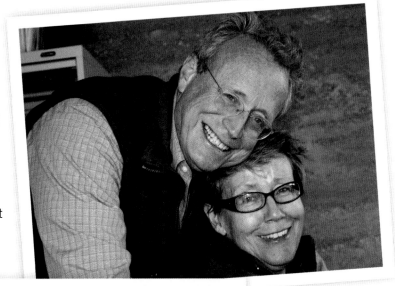

Stewart Francke

Detroit, Michigan

I was diagnosed with leukemia at the age of 39, had a bone marrow transplant at 40, and every breath since has been a gift.

On the day before Thanksgiving in 1998, I was given extreme unction, part of the Catholic Church's last rites. My nearness to death actually helped illuminate the rules for living that I felt compelled to pass along to my kids, ages 4 and 2 at the time, should I not make it home.

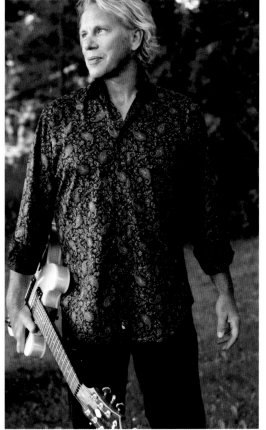

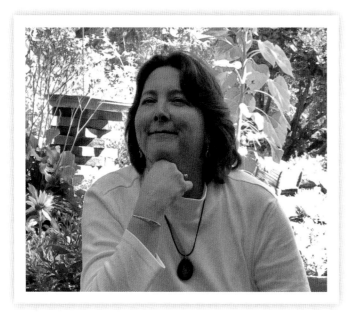

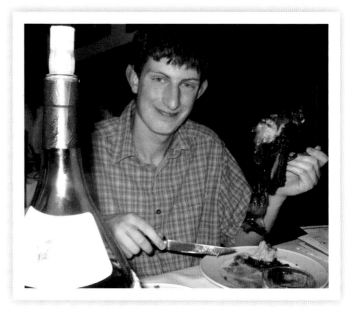

Sandi Duncan

La Crescenta, California

I now have the time to explore my creativity in all its expressions. I've gotten back into photography, and I spend more time in nature by taking day trips for photo outings. Another avenue of creative expression I've been very involved with is drumming. For years, I've participated in recreational drum circles, and I found that drumming really helped me when I was going through chemotherapy. It's not only fun, but it also relieves stress and is amazingly healing.

I've since trained to be a drum circle facilitator, and I now lead drum circles at the local Wellness Community Center for cancer patients and their caregivers. Drumming makes people happy, and being able to help others feel better is very rewarding. I'm coming up on my fourth year in remission, and I feel great!

Jake Silberg

New Jersey

My cancer experience is bookended by two trips to a hilltop hospital in Rome. On the first trip, I was 14 and supposed to be on vacation. Instead, I spent 28 days in a hospital, unable to eat or talk with my roommates. I was only able to wonder when life would go back to normal.

Two years later, I returned to that tiny room where I'd been told, "You have cancer." I thought back on everything I'd struggled through during the time between—chemotherapy, hair loss, and isolation. I reflected on the joy of each cancer-free scan and how lucky I was to be healthy when so many kids were still in treatment. I promised to cherish that gift. That night, I ate the most delicious Italian food. I had waited two years for it, and I will remember it always.

Glenda Goodwin

Atlanta, Georgia

The best part of "after cancer" is getting back to feeling exactly like you did before cancer. During my illness, I didn't think that was ever going to be possible.

This photo is from my daughter's wedding last September, and my son gets married next. To live to see both of them marry and be two of the most wonderful young adults is amazing!

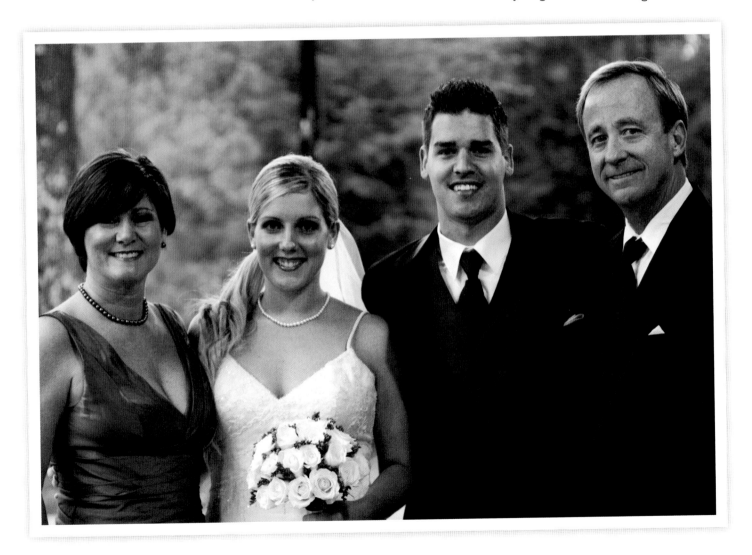

Annabel Weil

New York

Life is different after cancer because my mom, Katy, feels like she can do anything. She can publish a book. She can make a movie. She can follow her dreams. It's almost like life got better after cancer.

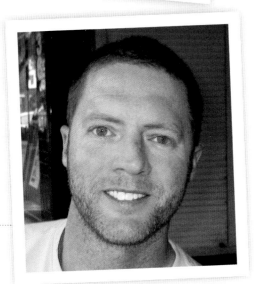

Buck Usher

Seattle, Washington

Life is different after cancer because my priorities have completely reversed. Before, I was motivated by my career and tended to neglect my personal life. Now, I put my life first. I take the time to go on vacations and enjoy my friends and family.

When one is faced with death, you suddenly realize what matters and what doesn't. Though I wouldn't wish cancer on anyone, it was probably the best thing to happen to me. It reminded me that you only live once, and you must make the most of your life while you can.

Michele Siegrist

Valdosta, Georgia

I was diagnosed with leukemia in July 2009 at age 18. In December 2009, I finished my chemotherapy treatments and was able to start my sophomore year of college the following January.

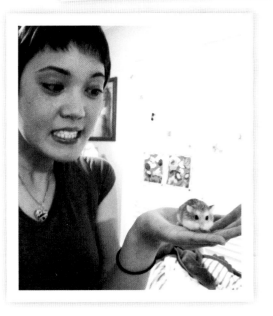

My journey through cancer has been such a blessing! Although it was life threatening, it was absolutely eye opening. I see life with a whole new perspective. I'm so much more thankful, even for the little things, which is what my picture kind of shows. The littlest things bring joy to my life. My journey is not over, though, as I still need a bone marrow transplant. I am ready for whatever comes next. I'm so thankful for what has happened in my life in the last nine months.

Jack Leggett

Mission Viejo, California

At first, I would have written about the side effects of prostate surgery. Now, I realize the more important change is that I am more present with my family in my daily life, grateful for the time I have, knowing I could have been out of time.

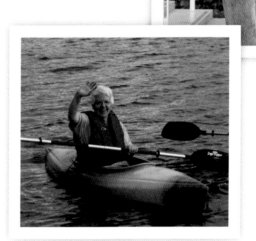

Pat Jenkins

Bangor, Maine

Shortly after chemotherapy and radiation were completed, I experienced my first time in a kayak. I find that I'm willing to try new things, and most important, I avoid stressing over the small stuff, or even the big stuff.

I recently had my wallet stolen with all of my identification and credit and debit cards. In the past, I would have gone ballistic. Now, as unpleasant as it was, I'm able to just remind myself that there are much worse things that can happen. I'm alive, relatively healthy, and have a wonderful family. How can I not be happy?

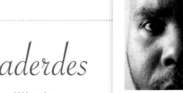

Rick Meaderdes

North Aurora, Illinois

I have an intense appreciation of life. I went on my first airplane ride and cruise. I've also learned how to ride a motorcycle. And I am glad to be here to welcome my fourth grandchild into the world.

Michael Lamanna

Chicago, Illinois

After cancer, I was inspired to build my dream world. We only have one life, and after going through this experience, I realized that I wanted to maximize my potential and make my one life as satisfying as possible. To me, that means continuing and creating rich relationships with others.

I was completely touched by my family and friends and wouldn't have survived this experience mentally or physically if it weren't for them. They made the difference for me, and now I want to make the difference for others.

Ron Ball

Annandale, Virginia

I quit smoking 14 years before I was diagnosed with stage IV tongue cancer, which spread to my neck, lung, and lymph nodes. It is currently a stage IV cancer, but I'm now more focused than ever before.

I do yoga, meditation, weightlifting, and endurance bicycling. An avid environmentalist, I commute 35 miles daily and will be amongst the first to get a Chevy Volt.

I wanted to live to see my son graduate high school and get into college. He got himself into an upstate New York "Little Ivy" with hard work and determination.

My life is full. I work with the severely mentally ill, which helps keep things in perspective. I'm reminded that the only love I feel is the love I give. Thank you for this opportunity.

Michelle Hastings

Phoenix, Arizona

Life is different now because I'm an active driver in my own life rather than a sedentary, passive passenger. I make things happen; I don't wait for them to happen.

Before cancer, I was a mom, wife, daughter, sister, and friend. Now, I am still all those things, but I get to add "colon cancer butt-kicker" to that list of titles.

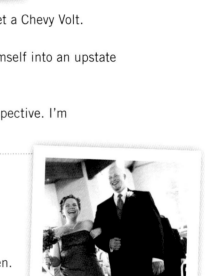

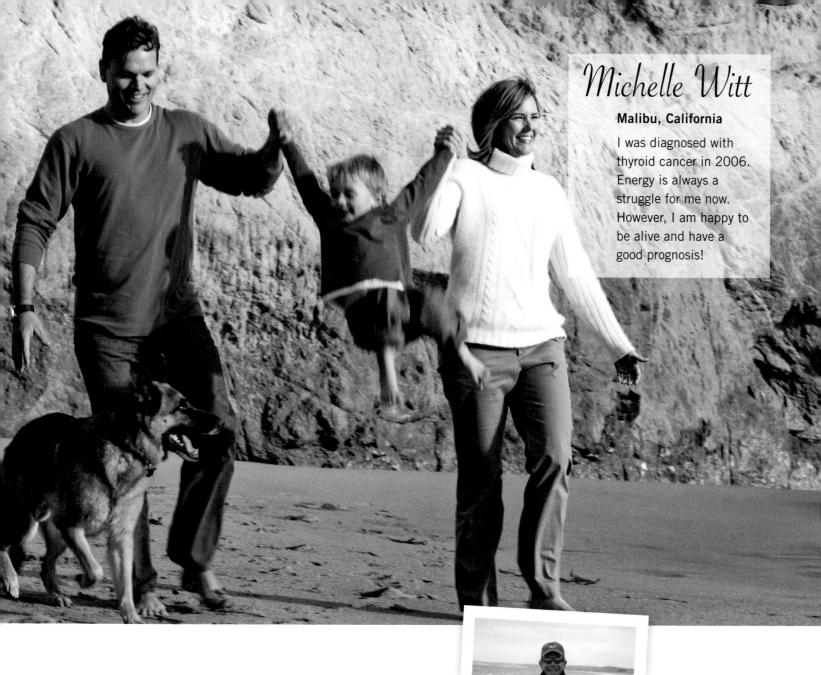

Michelle Witt

Malibu, California

I was diagnosed with thyroid cancer in 2006. Energy is always a struggle for me now. However, I am happy to be alive and have a good prognosis!

Richard Zuckerman

San Francisco, California

Never has the beach felt so magnificent!

Dick LaVine

New York, New York

In 2004, at age 67, I was diagnosed with myxofibrosarcoma of the right shoulder. Massive surgery removed the tumor along with my trapezius muscle and the top of the scapula and triceps.

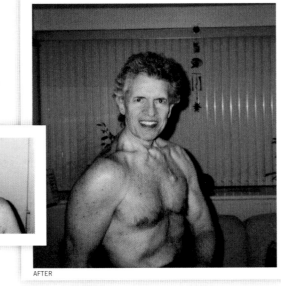

BEFORE

Five years later, I owe my life and vibrant, cancer-free health to the skill and compassion of my medical team and the love of my wife and friends. My wife and I are amateur Argentine tango dancers, and I am also a musician.

AFTER

I had four basic physical goals in mind for my intensive rehabilitation: to be able to dance in tango embrace position, to regain the dexterity necessary to play my instrument, to maintain my cardiovascular and strength levels, and to be as pain-free as possible without medication. I have wildly exceeded my goals.

Jennifer Bennette

Scottsdale, Arizona

I moved back to hot Arizona to be near my family and close friends. I am raising my two boys, Hunter (right) and Cooper, on my own. I started a jewelry business celebrating cancer survivors. Here I am at Relay For Life® with my kids!

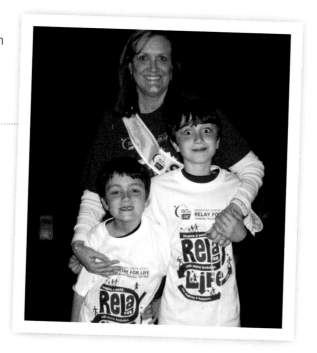

Leah Del Percio

New York

Cancer taught me to cherish every moment of my life and maintain a positive outlook in any and all situations, no matter how bad things may seem. It also taught me how strong, resilient, and determined I can be.

Hodgkin disease was diagnosed in my collarbone and chest at the age of 16, but I have been cancer free for nine years now. During those years, I ran multiple half marathons and graduated from high school, college, and law school. And I passed both the New York and New Jersey state bar exams on my first try!

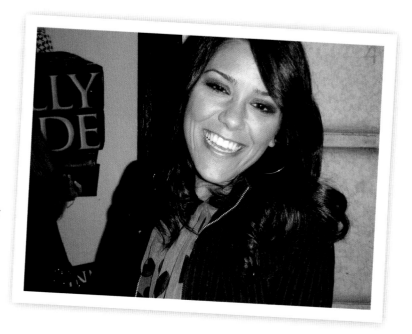

Though I wouldn't wish what I went through on anyone, I feel honored to be able to stand as living proof to other young cancer survivors that a cancer diagnosis is not the end of your dreams; it can be the beginning of them.

Jacki Donaldson

Gainesville, Florida

Life after cancer is better. I stress less. My love is deeper. My little boys are more precious. Family is number one. My hair is more stylish, eating is cleaner, fitness is fine-tuned, and my body is stronger. My job is a blessing. All the teeny, tiny moments of each day are, well, better.

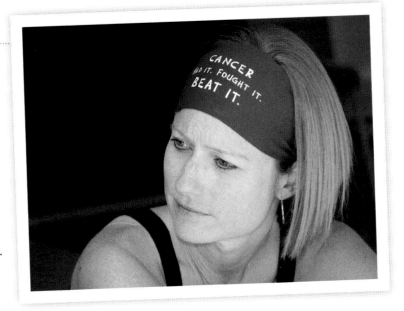

Elias Pietro Floris
Italy

Now, I know he's the bravest boy in the world.

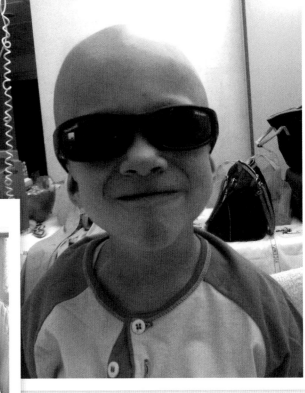

Heidi Floyd
Indiana

My life is in an entirely different place since I was diagnosed. I was pregnant with my son, Noah, when I went through chemotherapy. He and his sisters were the reason I got up every morning and fought through the difficulties. They make every day worthwhile. Although our family had a difficult journey, we are wiser and more compassionate on this side of the cancer experience. There isn't a day that passes that I don't thank God for my family, my friends, and my world.

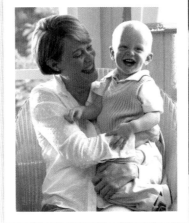

Nas Sarygulova
New York, New York

Before cancer, I did not like wearing the color red. Now, after breast cancer, red is the only color I wear. It's the color of life, joy, and radiance!

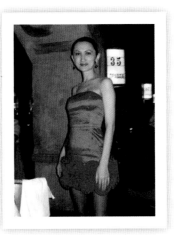

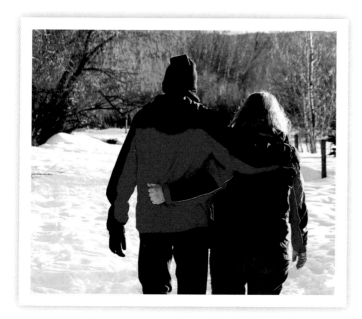

Christina Geller

Bozeman, Montana

This photo shows my mother, Barbara, and my younger brother, Jack, on a hike a little less than five years after she beat cancer. Life after cancer has definitely redefined our relationships with our mother and father. We're much more appreciative of the time we get to spend with our parents and the hugs and kisses she gives us.

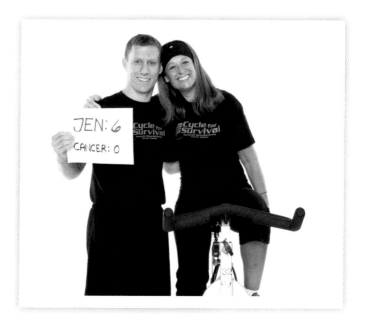

Jennifer Goodman Linn

New York, New York

I am a six-time cancer survivor and have been living with this disease for the past five years. I have slogged through five major abdominal surgeries and countless rounds of chemotherapy. I don't call myself a survivor but rather a "liver," someone who might have cancer, but doesn't allow cancer to have them. I have learned to find joy in the day-to-day and have realized how life can truly change on a dime.

Lindsay Kandra

Portland, Oregon

The things that used to matter don't matter anymore. And the things that used to not matter mean the world to me.

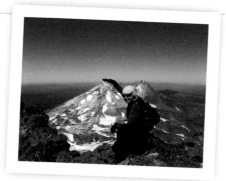

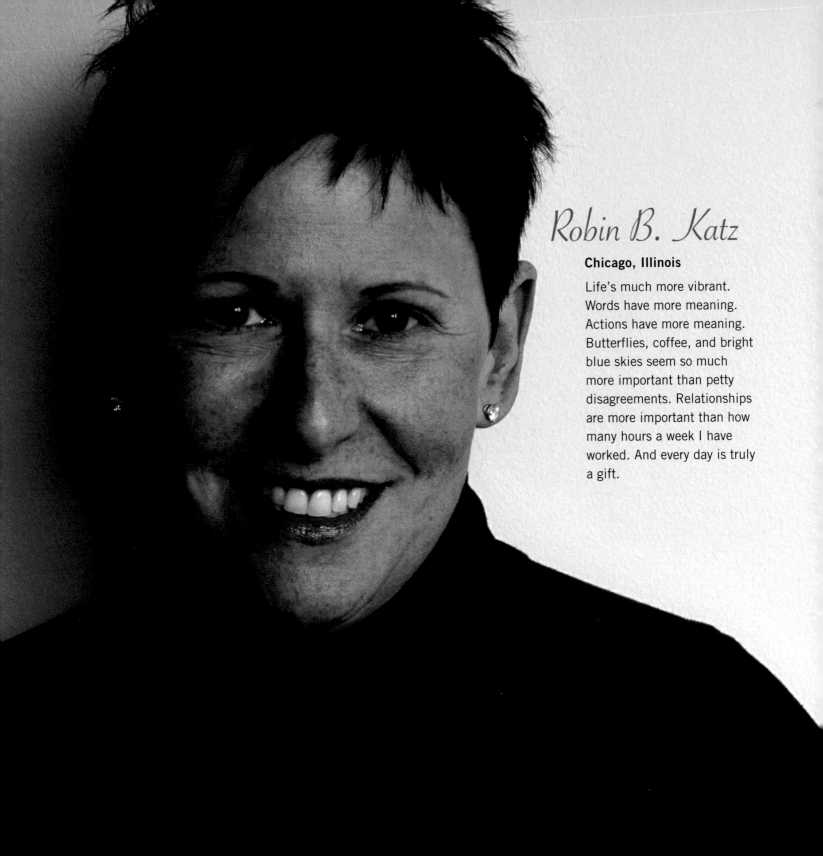

Robin B. Katz

Chicago, Illinois

Life's much more vibrant. Words have more meaning. Actions have more meaning. Butterflies, coffee, and bright blue skies seem so much more important than petty disagreements. Relationships are more important than how many hours a week I have worked. And every day is truly a gift.

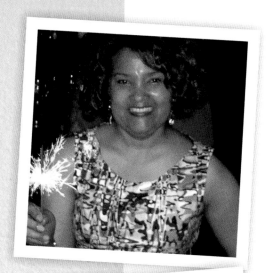

Debra Garrett

San Antonio, Texas

My experience with breast cancer has taught me to be bold—to seek a new career, to take a helicopter ride to a glacier, to fly in a floatplane. To soar and take others with me.

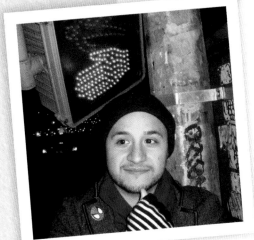

Pasquale Ricotta

New York, New York

Life after cancer is a lot different than people may think. It alters your state of mind, keeps you grounded and more in touch with reality. It's made me a little more cynical and distant at times, but one positive change is that it makes me appreciate how beautiful a day can really be.

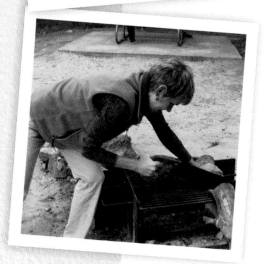

Lisa C. Kiewra

Pedernales Falls, Texas

Cancer is an invitation to seize the day. Since my breast cancer diagnosis, I try to do more of what I loved to do before. This includes immersing myself in nature in the company of good friends. In this picture, I am sawing logs for our campfire in central Texas. Being outside is an antidote for all that ails me!

MiMi Olsson

Attleboro, Massachusetts

Carly (on the far right) is a mesenchymal chondrosarcoma survivor and champion dancer! Living with chronic neuropathic pain does not slow her down. She is living life—not on the sidelines, but right up front.

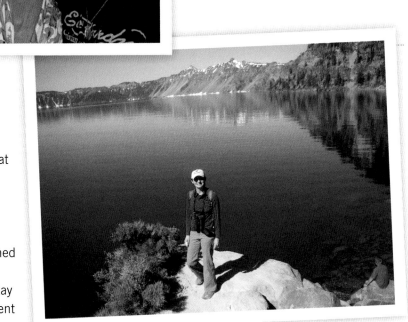

Heidi Brenke

Arizona

Love is deeper, and moments of beauty are right now.

Laura diZerega

San Luis Obispo, California

I was diagnosed with non-Hodgkin lymphoma at age 39 in July 2008. This photo was taken in July 2009 when we were celebrating my husband's birthday.

Everything is sweeter after cancer. I have learned so much, and I am grateful for it. But that doesn't mean it wasn't very scary at times. I stay focused on the incredible blessing of the present moment. I don't worry about the things I can't control. I tell my loved ones how very much I love them. And I am in awe of my doctors and nurses who do the bravest work of all.

Beth Silverman

Baltimore, Maryland

I never expected to get diagnosed with breast cancer at the age of 26. Cancer tried to steal everything from me: my hair, my breasts, my boyfriend, my career, and the feeling that nothing in life would ever be harder to do than fight cancer. WELL, I WAS WRONG!

In the last two years, I have rappelled off skyscrapers, kayaked class III rapids in Colorado, dangled from large rocks in Moab, Utah, and trekked through the Canadian Rockies. Cancer may not play fair, but I only play to win. I have never felt more alive.

All that I do now, I do on my terms. To honor the 51 friends I've buried to this disease and the 28 million people living with cancer, I live fully, love deeply, and laugh a whole heck of a lot.

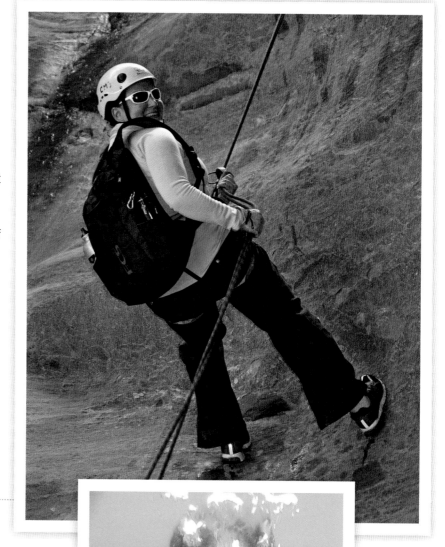

Miriam R. Robbins

New York, New York

When I was diagnosed with Hodgkin disease almost 20 years ago, I was determined that as soon as I was physically able, I was going to learn how to scuba dive. Scuba diving was something I had wanted to do since I was 8 years old. And I did.

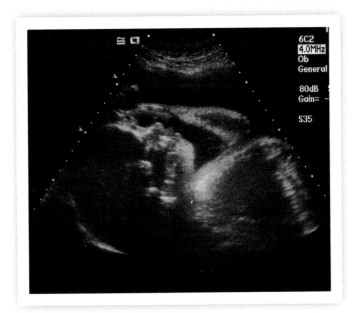

J.M. Cassidy

New York, New York

Little things mean a whole lot more. Family comes first. Prior to my diagnosis, a new family wasn't even a picture on the horizon. After cancer, things have changed. I'm truly experiencing life, not just living it. I've gladly taken on the responsibilities of survivorship. I'm helping others by providing support to both friends and strangers throughout diagnosis and treatment, and I am guiding friends and family in how to make a difference in the lives of those affected by cancer, especially pediatric cancer.

My motto: "It's remarkably easy to make a difference."

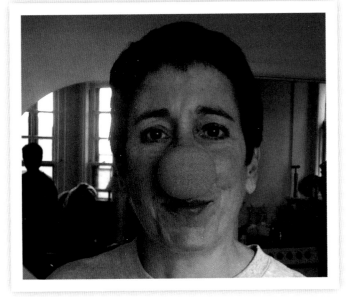

Debra Goodman

New York, New York

Life is easier.

I've already mentally come to terms with my mortality, and I am ready to make the most of every day.

Okay, most days.

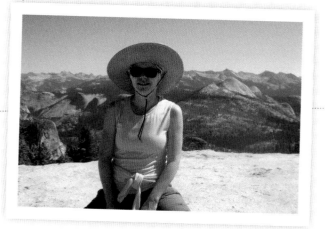

Susan Henry

Los Angeles, California

Sweeter. Easier. Better.

Surviving and Thriving After Cancer

From the AMERICAN CANCER SOCIETY

As you can see from reading the heartfelt entries in these pages, life *after cancer* is different for every person. In fact, life is transformed the moment a person hears the words "you have cancer," and nothing is ever the same again.

Many people who have survived cancer report that the time after treatment was the most difficult for them emotionally. Most people find themselves dealing with a range of feelings, sometimes all happening at once. Follow-up visits, anniversary dates of your cancer diagnosis, movies about cancer—any of these can stir up strong emotions. Anything that reminds you of your cancer experience can make you feel sad, anxious, or angry.

Surviving and thriving

Only a few decades ago, the prognosis (outlook) for people facing cancer was not nearly as favorable as it is today. During the 1970s, about one of two people diagnosed with cancer survived at least five years. Now, more than two of three survive that long and longer. Today there are more than 12 million cancer survivors in the United States alone.

Now that more people are surviving cancer, more attention than ever is focused on quality of life and the long-term outcomes of cancer survivors. Behavioral researchers are working to learn more about the problems survivors face. Some of these problems are medical, such as permanent side effects of treatment, the possibility of second cancers caused by treatment, and the need for long-term treatment and medical follow-up. Other problems are emotional or social challenges, like getting health insurance, discrimination by employers, relationship changes that may result from life-threatening illness, or learning to live with the possibility of cancer coming back.

Cancer was once a word that people were afraid to speak in public, and people rarely admitted to being a cancer survivor. Now, many celebrities and national leaders very openly discuss and share their cancer experiences. The view that cancer cannot be cured and the fears that have historically been attached to the disease are slowly changing.

Finding hope

Today cancer is not a death sentence. Cure rates continue to improve as new medicines and treatments are discovered. Some types of cancer have better prognoses (outlooks) than others but, overall, people with cancer are living longer.

Doctors cannot predict how long a person will live. They can only make an educated guess, based on what they have seen in other patients in similar situations. Even when a person's outlook is poor, new research discoveries and treatments that can control the disease can give hope. If a loved one has cancer, your continued love and support can also provide hope.

Regardless of the prognosis, this time is a chance to do things you've always wanted to do and to spend quality time with family and friends.

Keep the focus on what you can do rather than what you can't. Lead an active life and have a sense of purpose. These things help most people cope with cancer. It's not always possible to do things you did in the past, but there are usually ways to make each day count.

Making healthy choices

Think about your life before cancer. Were there things you did that might have made you less healthy? Maybe you drank too much, ate more than you needed, smoked, or didn't exercise very often. Maybe you kept your feelings bottled up, or maybe you let stressful things go on too long.

You can start making changes today that can have good effects for the rest of your life. You'll feel better and be healthier, too.

You can start by working on those things that bother you most. Get help with the changes that are harder for you. For instance, if you are thinking about quitting smoking and need help, call the American Cancer Society at **800-227-2345**.

Eating healthy

Eating right can be hard to do, during and after cancer treatment. Treatment may change your sense of taste. You may have a sick stomach. You may not feel like eating. You may even lose weight when you don't want to. On the other hand, some people gain weight even without eating more. This can be upsetting, too.

If you are losing weight or have taste problems, do the best you can with eating and know that these problems will get better. You may want to ask your doctor or nurse to see a dietitian who can give you ideas on how to deal with some of these side effects. You may also find it helps to eat small meals every two to three hours until you feel better.

One of the best things you can do after treatment is put healthy eating habits into place. Try to eat two and a half cups or more of vegetables and fruits each day. Choose whole grain foods instead of white flour and sugars. Cut back on red meat and processed meats, such as hot dogs, deli meats, and bacon. If you drink alcohol, limit yourself to no more than one drink a day for women or two drinks a day for men. And don't forget to get regular exercise. A good diet and regular exercise will help you stay at a healthy weight and give you more energy.

Dealing with fatigue, work, and exercise

Fatigue or feeling very tired is very common in people with cancer. This tired feeling is not the same as the tiredness you might have at the end of a very busy day. It is a "bone-weary" feeling that doesn't get better with rest. For some, this fatigue lasts a long time after treatment.

It can be hard to be active when you feel tired all the time. But being active can help reduce your fatigue. Studies have shown that patients who follow an exercise program feel better and cope better, too.

If you were sick or on bed rest during treatment, it's normal to have lost some of your fitness, endurance, and muscle strength. Exercise can help you make your muscles strong, and can help fight fatigue. It can also help the depressed feeling that sometimes comes with being so tired.

Your exercise program should fit your needs. An older person who has never been very active may not be able to do the same amount of exercise as a 20-year-old. If you haven't been active in a few years but can still get around, you may want to think about starting with short walks.

Talk with your doctor or nurse before starting. Let them know about your plans. And try to find an exercise buddy so that you're not doing it alone. Having family or friends join you in a new exercise program can give you that extra boost of support to keep you going when the push just isn't there. If you are very tired, though, you will need to be sure you get some rest. It's hard for some people to allow themselves to rest when they are used to working all day or taking care of a home and family. It's okay to rest when you need to.

Exercise can improve your health:

- It improves your heart and circulation.
- It makes your muscles stronger.
- It helps fatigue.
- It lowers anxiety and depression.
- It makes you feel happier.
- It helps you feel better about yourself.

And we know that exercise plays a role in preventing some cancers. The American Cancer Society says adults should get 150 minutes of moderate physical activity or 75 minutes of vigorous physical activity, or a combination of the two, each week. Children and teens should get 60 minutes of moderate physical activity each day with vigorous physical activity three days each week.

Dealing with emotions

Once your treatment ends, you may find yourself filled with emotions. This happens to a lot of people.

You may have been going through so much since diagnosis that you could only focus on getting through your treatment. Now you may find that you think about your own death or the effect of your cancer on your family. You may also begin to think about your relationship with your spouse or partner.

This is a time when you need people you can turn to for strength and comfort. This support can come from family, friends, cancer support groups, church groups, online support groups, or counselors.

Seeking support

Almost everyone who has been through cancer feels better if he or she gets some type of support. What's best for you depends on you. Some people feel safe in groups; others would rather talk in an informal setting, such as church. Others may feel more at ease talking with a close friend or counselor. Whatever your source of strength or comfort, make sure you have a place to go with your concerns. The American Cancer Society Cancer Survivors Network® (csn.cancer.org) offers a community for cancer survivors, families, and friends to share experiences. CancerCare® and the National Coalition for Cancer Survivorship are other organizations that offer support programs for cancer survivors. For more information about these and other organizations, see the Resource Guide, starting on the next page.

The cancer journey can feel very lonely. You don't need to go it alone. Your friends and family may feel shut out if you decide not to include them. Let them in—and let in those who you feel may help. If you aren't sure who can help, call the American Cancer Society at **800-227-2345** anytime, day or night.

You can't change the fact that you have had cancer.
What you *can* change is how you live the rest of your life.

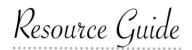
Resource Guide

AMERICAN CANCER SOCIETY SUPPORT PROGRAMS AND SERVICES

American Cancer Society
Toll-free: 800-227-2345
Web site: cancer.org

The American Cancer Society is the nationwide, community-based voluntary health organization dedicated to eliminating cancer as a major health problem by preventing cancer, saving lives, and diminishing suffering from cancer through research, education, advocacy, and service. Headquartered in Atlanta, Georgia, the Society has 12 chartered Divisions, more than 900 local offices nationwide, and a presence in more than 5,100 communities.

The American Cancer Society provides educational materials, information, and patient services to help people with cancer and their loved ones understand cancer, manage their lives through treatment and recovery, and find the emotional support they need. A comprehensive resource for all your cancer-related questions, the Society can also put you in touch with community resources in your area.

And best of all, our help is free.

Cancer Action Network™ (ACS CAN) is all about ensuring that fighting cancer is a top priority for our lawmakers. When constituents demand that legislators make fighting cancer a priority, they make a difference. All ACS CAN members are notified of cancer-related issues pending in government agencies. They are also notified when critical cancer issues are heading for a vote or are in danger of being ignored by our lawmakers.
Web site: acscan.org

The Cancer Survivors Network® comprises a community of cancer survivors, families, and friends. All have been touched by cancer and want to share their experiences, strength, and hope. Only those who have been there can truly understand. The Web site is completely non-commercial and provides a private, secure way to find and communicate with others to share similar interests and experiences. Members control access to personal information.
Web site: csn.cancer.org

Look Good…Feel Better® is a free, community-based program that teaches beauty techniques to female cancer patients to help them manage the appearance-related side effects of cancer treatment. The program is open to all women with cancer who are undergoing chemotherapy, radiation, or other forms of treatment. The thousands of volunteer beauty professionals who support Look Good…Feel Better are trained and certified by the Personal Care Products Council Foundation, the American Cancer Society, and the Professional Beauty Association I National Cosmetology Association at local, statewide, and national workshops.
Web site: lookgoodfeelbetter.org

The **American Cancer Society Patient Navigator Program** helps patients, families, and caregivers navigate the many systems needed during the cancer journey. Trained Patient Navigators at cancer treatment centers link those dealing with cancer to needed programs and resources. The "navigator" is a friendly, experienced, and approachable American Cancer Society staff person who helps patients have a better experience while they are receiving care.

Reach to Recovery® has helped people (female and male) cope with their breast cancer experience. This experience begins when someone is faced with the possibility of a breast cancer diagnosis and continues throughout the entire period that breast cancer remains a personal concern. Reach to Recovery volunteers offer understanding, support, and hope because they themselves have survived breast cancer and gone on to live normal, productive lives.

The **Road to Recovery®** program provides transportation to and from treatment for people who have cancer who do not have a ride or are unable to drive themselves. Volunteer drivers donate their time and the use of their cars so that patients can receive the life-saving treatments they need. Call **800-227-2345** to find out if Road to Recovery is available in your community.

Hope Lodge® offers cancer patients and their families a free, temporary place to stay when their best hope for effective treatment may be in another city. Having to travel away from home to get care can place an extra emotional and financial burden on patients and caregivers during an already challenging time. Currently, there are 31 Hope Lodge locations throughout the United States. Accommodations and eligibility requirements may vary by location, and room availability is first come, first served. Call **800-227-2345** to find out if there is a Hope Lodge location in your treatment area.

I Can Cope® is an educational program for adults facing cancer—either personally, or as a friend or family caregiver. I Can Cope cancer education classes can help patients and their loved ones learn about cancer and how to take care of themselves. I Can Cope classes can help dispel cancer myths by presenting straightforward information and answers to cancer-related questions on a variety of topics. For more information about I Can Cope classes in your area, call **800-227-2345**, or visit the Web site: cancer.org

The **Man to Man®** program helps men cope with prostate cancer by offering community-based education and support for patients and their family members. A core component of the program is the self-help and/or support group. Volunteers organize free monthly meetings where speakers and participants learn about and discuss information about prostate cancer, treatment, side effects, and how to cope with prostate cancer and its treatment. Programs, services, and activities vary, depending on the location. A six-page Man to Man newsletter is offered three times a year, distributed through local and regional American Cancer Society offices. Call **800-227-2345** for more information or to find a Man to Man program in your area.

Relay For Life®, the American Cancer Society's signature event, is an overnight experience designed to bring together those who have been touched by cancer. At Relay, people from within the community gather to celebrate survivors, remember those lost to cancer, and to fight back against this disease. Relay participants help raise money and awareness to support the American Cancer Society in its lifesaving mission to eliminate cancer as a major health issue.
Web site: relayforlife.org

The **"tlc" Tender Loving Care®** magalog is the American Cancer Society's catalog and magazine for women. It offers helpful articles and a line of products made for women with cancer. Products include wigs, hairpieces, breast forms, hats, turbans, mastectomy bras, and swimwear. The "tlc" mission is to make these hard-to-find products affordable and readily available in the privacy of your own home. All proceeds from product sales go back into the American Cancer Society's programs and services for patients and survivors. To order products or catalogs, call 800-850-9445, or visit "tlc" online at www.tlcdirect.org.

GENERAL CANCER RESOURCES

Association of Community Cancer Centers
11600 Nebel Street, Suite 201
Rockville, MD 20852-2557
Telephone: 301-984-9496
Fax: 301-770-1949
Web site: www.accc-cancer.org

The Association of Community Cancer Centers (ACCC) was founded to give oncology practitioners in the community a voice in the national oncology forum. ACCC includes more than 700 medical centers, hospitals, and cancer programs. The Web site features a searchable database of cancer centers listed by state (www.accc-cancer.org/membership_directory), Internet resources for cancer survivors (www.accc-cancer.org/education/education-cancersurvivorship-relatedlinks.asp), and other useful information.

CancerCare®
275 Seventh Avenue, 22nd Floor
New York, NY 10001
Cancer Care Counseling
Toll-free: 800-813-HOPE (800-813-4673)
Telephone: 212-712-8400
Fax: 212-719-0263
E-mail: info@cancercare.org
Web site: www.cancercare.org

CancerCare is a nonprofit social service agency that provides counseling and guidance to help cancer patients and their families and friends cope with the impact of cancer. CancerCare offers support groups; teleconferences for patients, friends, and family members; workshops, seminars and clinics; a newsletter, and other publications. CancerCare also provides a financial assistance program for constituents in New Jersey, New York, and Connecticut. The CancerCare Web site has detailed information on cancer, cancer treatment, clinical trials, services, and links to other cancer-related sites.

Cancer Hope Network
2 North Road, Suite A
Chester, NJ 07930
Toll-free: 800-552-4366
Telephone: 908-879-4039
Fax: 908-879-6518
E-mail: info@cancerhopenetwork.org
Web site: www.cancerhopenetwork.org

Cancer Hope Network is a nonprofit organization that provides free and confidential one-on-one support to cancer patients and their families. Their core offering is to match cancer patients or family members with trained volunteers who have themselves undergone and recovered from a similar cancer experience. Matches with support volunteers can be requested by calling the toll-free number or submitting the request online.

Cancer Research Institute
National Headquarters
One Exchange Plaza
55 Broadway, Suite 1802
New York, NY 10006
Toll-free: 800-992-2623 (800-99-CANCER)
Telephone: 212-688-7515
Fax: 212-832-9376
Web site: www.cancerresearch.org

The Cancer Research Institute (CRI) is dedicated exclusively to the support and coordination of laboratory and clinical efforts that will lead to the immunological treatment, control, and prevention of cancer. CRI has supported the work of nearly 3,000 researchers. The organization provides public information on cancer immunology and cancer treatment, helps locate immunotherapy clinical trials, and offers informational booklets on cancer.

Cancer Support Community
1050 17th Street, NW
Washington, DC 20036
Toll-free: 888-793-9355
Telephone: 202-659-9709
Fax: 202-974-7999
Web site: www.cancersupportcommunity.org

In June 2011, Gilda's Club Worldwide and The Wellness Community officially merged to become the Cancer Support Community (CSC). The mission of the Cancer Support Community is to ensure that all people impacted by cancer are empowered by knowledge, strengthened by action, and sustained by community. CSC provides the highest quality emotional and social support through a network of local affiliates and satellite locations. Visit their Web site to find a community-based center in your area.

CaringBridge.org
1715 Yankee Doodle Road, Suite 301
Eagan, MN 55121
Telephone: 651-452-7940
Fax: 651-681-7115
Web site: www.caringbridge.org

CaringBridge is a nonprofit organization that provides free Web sites to connect people experiencing a significant health challenge with their family and friends. CaringBridge Web sites offer a personal and private space to communicate and show support, saving time and emotional energy when health matters most. The Web sites are easy to create and use. Authors add health updates and photos to share their story while visitors leave messages of love, hope, and compassion in the guestbook.

LIVESTRONG Survivor Care Program
2201 E. Sixth Street
Austin, TX 78702
Toll-free: 866-236-8820
Web site: www.livestrong.org

The LIVESTRONG Survivor Care Program helps anyone affected by cancer—whether the individual is a cancer patient, family member, or friend of someone diagnosed. LIVESTRONG helps people understand their options, what to expect, and questions to ask. One-on-one support is provided all along the way.

National Cancer Institute
6116 Executive Boulevard, Room 3036A
Bethesda, MD 20892-8322
Toll-free: 800-4-CANCER (800-422-6237)
TTY (Text Telephone): 800-332-8615
Telephone: 301-496-5583
Fax: 301-402-5874
Web site: www.cancer.gov

The National Cancer Institute provides information on cancer research, diagnosis, and treatment to patients and health care providers. Callers are automatically connected to the office serving their region. The service offers free publications and the opportunity to speak directly with a cancer specialist who is trained to provide accurate information on treatment and prevention of cancer and to make appropriate referrals.

CancerTrials
Web site: www.cancer.gov/clinicaltrials

Maintained by the National Cancer Institute, this site offers information about ongoing cancer clinical trials and explanations of what a trial is and what is involved. Links are provided to allow users to search for clinical trials by city, state, and type of cancer from a database of more than 8,000 clinical trials in progress. Other popular links on this site include the "Dictionary of Cancer Terms" and the "NCI Drug Dictionary."

National Coalition for Cancer Survivorship
1010 Wayne Avenue, Suite 770
Silver Spring, MD 20910
Toll-free: 888-650-9127
Telephone: 301-650-9127
Fax: 301-565-9670
E-mail: info@canceradvocacy.org
Web site: www.canceradvocacy.org

The National Coalition for Cancer Survivorship (NCCS) is a network of independent organizations working in the area of cancer survivorship and support. Its primary goal is to generate a nationwide awareness of cancer survivorship. NCCS serves as an information clearinghouse and as an advocacy group.

National Alliance for Caregiving
4720 Montgomery Lane, 5th Floor
Bethesda, MD 20814
E-mail: info@caregiving.org
Web site: www.caregiving.org

The National Alliance for Caregiving is a nonprofit coalition of national organizations focusing on issues of family caregiving. Alliance members include grassroots organizations, professional associations, service organizations, disease-specific organizations, a government agency, and corporations. The Alliance was created to conduct research, do policy analysis, develop national programs, increase public awareness of family caregiving issues, work to strengthen state and local caregiving coalitions, and represent the U.S. caregiving community internationally. Recognizing that family caregivers provide important societal and financial contributions toward maintaining the well-being of those they care for, the Alliance's mission is to be the objective national resource on family caregiving with the goal of improving the quality of life for families and care recipients.

National Family Caregivers Association
10400 Connecticut Avenue, Suite 500
Kensington, MD 20895-3944
Toll-free: 800-896-3650
Telephone: 301-942-6430
Fax: 301-942-2302
E-mail: info@thefamilycaregiver.org
Web site: www.nfcacares.org

The National Family Caregivers Association (NFCA) educates, supports, empowers, and speaks up for the more than 50 million Americans who care for loved ones with a chronic illness or disability or the frailties of old age. NFCA reaches across the boundaries of diagnoses, relationships, and life stages to help transform family caregivers' lives by removing barriers to health and well-being. It provides information, education, public awareness, and advocacy.

RESOURCES FOR CHILDREN AND ADOLESCENTS

Cancer Really Sucks
Web site: www.cancerreallysucks.org

Cancer Really Sucks is an Internet-only resource designed for teens by teens who have loved ones facing cancer.

Cancercare for Kids
275 Seventh Avenue, Floor 22
New York, NY 10001
Toll-free Line: 800-813-HOPE (800-813-4673)
E-mail: info@cancercare.org
Web site: www.cancercareforkids.org

Cancercare for Kids is an online support program for teens with a parent, sibling, or other family member who has cancer. The toll-free number is also for anyone who has cancer or has a loved one with cancer.

CLIMB®
The Children's Treehouse Foundation
50 South Steele Street, Suite 810
Denver, CO 80209
Telephone: 303-322-1202
Fax: 303-322-3676
E-mail: achildstreehouse@aol.com
Web site: www.childrenstreehousefdn.org

CLIMB (Children's Lives Include Moments of Bravery) is a support group program for children of adult cancer patients. CLIMB is a program that helps children find the courage to deal with cancer in their families. The program helps normalize feelings of sadness, anxiety, fear, and anger of the children, while stimulating improved communications between the children and their parents. CLIMB is a program of The Children's Treehouse Foundation and is offered in medical treatment facilities throughout the nation.

KidsCope
2045 Peachtree Road, Suite 150
Atlanta, GA 30309
Web site: www.kidscope.org

KidsCope is an Internet-only resource for children and families. Its mission is to help children and families understand the effects of cancer or chemotherapy on a loved one, to provide suggestions for coping, and to develop innovative programs and materials that communicate a message of hope. The Web site offers resources, including a comic book for children about chemotherapy (Kemo Shark) and a video for kids about a mom with breast cancer.

Kids Konnected
26071 Merit Circle, Suite 103
Laguna Hills, CA 92653
Toll-free: 800-899-2866
Telephone: 949-582-5443
Email: info@kidskonnected.org
Web site: www.kidskonnected.org

Kids Konnected is a national organization that offers groups and programs for children who have a parent with cancer. They provide information, referrals to local services, a newsletter, and grief workshops.

ADDITIONAL RESOURCES

Alliance of State Pain Initiatives
University of Wisconsin School of Medicine and Public Health
1300 University Avenue, Room 4720
Madison, WI 53706
Telephone: 608-262-0978
Fax: 608-265-4014
E-mail: trc@mailplus.wisc.edu
Web site: www.trc.wisc.edu

The Alliance of State Pain Initiatives (ASPI) is a national network of interdisciplinary, state-based organizations dedicated to transforming the culture of pain care. State Pain Initiatives are typically volunteer groups composed of nurses, physicians, pharmacists, social workers, psychologists, patient advocates, and representatives of clergy, government, and higher education who are working to improve the care of persons with pain. This network promotes the relief of cancer pain through advocacy and education by providing information for patients about pain management and developing educational, advocacy, and institutional improvement programs.

American Academy of Physical Medicine and Rehabilitation (for locating physiatrists)
330 North Wabash Avenue, Suite 2500
Chicago, IL 60611-7617
Telephone: 312-464-9700
Fax: 312-464-0227
E-mail: info@aapmr.org
Web site: www.aapmr.org

The American Academy of Physical Medicine and Rehabilitation is the national medical society representing more than 7,500 physicians who are specialists in the field of physical medicine and rehabilitation.

American Pain Foundation
201 N. Charles Street, Suite 710
Baltimore, MD 21201-4111
Toll-free: 888-615-PAIN (888-615-7246)
E-mail: info@painfoundation.org
Web site: www.painfoundation.org

The American Pain Foundation is an independent nonprofit organization serving people with pain through information, advocacy, and support. Their mission is to improve the quality of life of people with pain by raising public awareness, providing practical information, promoting research, and advocating to remove barriers and increase access to effective pain management.

American Physical Therapy Association
1111 North Fairfax Street
Alexandria, VA 22314-1488
Toll-free: 800-999-APTA (800-999-2782)
Fax: 703-684-7343
Web site: www.apta.org

The American Physical Therapy Association (APTA) is a national professional organization representing more than 72,000 members. The organization represents and promotes the profession of physical therapy and strives to further the profession's role in the prevention, diagnosis, and treatment of movement dysfunctions and the enhancement of the physical health and functional abilities of members of the public. Its goal is to foster advancements in physical therapy through practice, research, and education.

CancerConnection
P.O. Box 60452
Florence, MA 01062
Telephone: 413-586-1642
Web site: www.cancer-connection.org

CancerConnection is a community-based, nonprofit organization. Founded in 2000, it offers a haven where people living with cancer, their families, and their caregivers can learn how to cope with their changed lives and bodies and emotional turmoil by sharing strategies and resources. All offerings are free.

International Association of Laryngectomees
925B Peachtree Street NE, Suite 316
Atlanta, GA 30309
Toll-free: 866-425-3678
Web site: www.theial.com

The International Association of Laryngectomees (IAL) is a nonprofit voluntary organization composed of approximately 300 laryngectomee member clubs. The purpose of the IAL is to assist local clubs in their efforts toward total rehabilitation after laryngectomy. IAL programs include skills education for laryngectomees; a registry of alaryngeal (post-laryngectomy) speech instructors; the Voice Rehabilitation Institute, which trains laryngectomees and therapists; and educational materials.

Leukemia & Lymphoma Society
1311 Mamaroneck Avenue, Suite 310
White Plains, NY 10605
Toll-free: 800-955-4572
Telephone: 914-949-5213
Fax: 914-949-6691
E-mail: infocenter@lls.org
Web site: www.lls.org

The Leukemia & Lymphoma Society (LLS) is dedicated to the cure of leukemia, lymphoma, Hodgkin disease, and myeloma and to improving quality of life for patients and their families. Patient service programs and resources available through local chapters of the LLS include financial assistance, support groups, one-to-one volunteer visitors (in some chapters), patient education and information, and referral to local resources in the community.

National Association of Hospital Hospitality Houses, Inc.
44 Merrimon Avenue, 1st Floor
Asheville, NC 28801
Toll-free: 800-542-9730
Telephone: 828-253-1188
Fax: 828-542-9730
E-mail: helpinghomes@nahhh.org
Web site: www.nahhh.com

The National Association of Hospital Hospitality Houses, Inc. (NAHHH) provides information about hospital hospitality facilities, including Ronald McDonald Houses. These facilities provide lodging and other supportive services in a home-like environment, primarily for relatives of patients seeking medical treatment outside their own community. Services vary from facility to facility and are offered at little or no cost to the guests.

National Bone Marrow Transplant Link
20411 West 12 Mile Road, Suite 108
Southfield, MI 48076
Toll-free: 800-546-5268 (800-LINK-BMT)
Telephone: 248-358-1886
Fax: 248-358-1889
E-mail: info@nbmtlink.org
Web site: www.nbmtlink.org

The National Bone Marrow Transplant Link helps patients, caregivers, and families cope with the social and emotional challenges of bone marrow/stem cell transplant from diagnosis through survivorship by providing vital information and personalized support services. The Web site contains links to a BMT resource guide, a survivorship guide, and a caregivers' guide, among other materials. Resources for health care professionals are also available.

National Lymphedema Network
Latham Square
1611 Telegraph Avenue, Suite 111
Oakland, CA 94612-2138
Telephone: 510-208-3200
Fax: 510-208-3110
Web site: www.lymphnet.org

The National Lymphedema Network (NLN) is a nonprofit organization providing education and guidance to lymphedema patients, health care professionals, and the public by disseminating information on the prevention and management of primary and secondary lymphedema. The NLN is supported by tax-deductible donations and is a driving force behind the movement in the U.S. to standardize quality treatment for lymphedema patients nationwide. In addition, the NLN supports research into the causes and possible alternative treatments for this often incapacitating, long-neglected condition.

The Office on Women's Health
U.S. Department of Health and Human Services
8270 Willow Oaks Corporate Drive, Suite 101
Fairfax, VA 22031
Toll-free: 800-994-9662
Web site: www.womenshealth.gov

The Office on Women's Health (OWH) provides leadership to promote health equity for women and girls through sex- and gender-specific approaches. OWH achieves its mission and vision by developing innovative programs, educating health professionals, and motivating behavior change in consumers through the dissemination of health information. Its Web site offers a database of information on various women's health issues, including breast cancer. Documents accessible through this site include information from the National Cancer Institute, the Centers for Disease Control and Prevention, and several other government agencies.

Patient Advocate Foundation
700 Thimble Shoals Boulevard, Suite 200
Newport News, VA 23606
Toll-free: 800-532-5274
Fax: 757-873-8999
E-mail: help@patientadvocate.org
Web site: www.patientadvocate.org

Patient Advocate Foundation (PAF) is a national nonprofit organization that provides professional case management services to Americans with chronic, life threatening, and debilitating illnesses. PAF case managers, assisted by doctors and health care attorneys, serve as active liaisons between patient and insurer, employer, and/or creditor to resolve insurance, job retention, and/or debt crisis matters. Patient Advocate Foundation seeks to safeguard patients through effective mediation, ensuring access to care, maintenance of employment, and preservation of their financial stability.

Pharmaceutical Research and Manufacturers Association of America
950 F Street, NW
Washington, DC 20004
Telephone: 202-835-3400
Fax: 202-835-3414
Web site: www.phrma.org

The Pharmaceutical Research and Manufacturers of America (PhRMA) represents the country's leading pharmaceutical research and biotechnology companies, which are devoted to inventing medicines that allow patients to live longer, healthier, and more productive lives.

Partnership for Prescription Assistance
Toll-free Line: 888-4PPA-NOW (888-477-2669)
Web site: www.pparx.org

The Partnership for Prescription Assistance helps qualifying patients without prescription drug coverage get the medicines they need through the program that is right for them. The organization provides a Directory of Prescription Drug Patient Assistance Programs that contains information about how to make a request for assistance, what prescription medicines are covered, and basic eligibility criteria.

Self Help for Women with Breast or Ovarian Cancer
1501 Broadway, Suite 704A
New York, NY 10036
Toll-free/Breast Cancer: 866-891-2392
Toll-free/Ovarian Cancer: 866-537-4273
Telephone: 212-719-0364
Web site: www.sharecancersupport.org

Self Help for Women with Breast or Ovarian Cancer (SHARE) is a self-help organization that serves women who have been affected by breast cancer or ovarian cancer. Hotline volunteers are breast or ovarian cancer survivors. They provide information about breast cancer, emotional support, printed materials, and referrals to national organizations. Their Web site includes information on the hotlines and support programs in New York City. Spanish speaking staff are available.

Sisters Network® Inc.
8787 Woodway Drive, Suite 4206
Houston, TX 77063
Telephone: 713-781-0255
Toll-free: 866-781-1808
Fax: 713-780-8998
Web site: www.sistersnetworkinc.org

Sisters Network Inc. is a national African American breast cancer survivorship organization. This nonprofit organization is committed to increasing local and national attention on the devastating impact that breast cancer has in the African American Community.

United Ostomy Associations of America, Inc.
P.O. Box 66
Fairview, TN 37062-0066
Toll-free: 800-826-0826
E-mail: info@uoaa.org
Web site: www.uoa.org

The United Ostomy Associations of America, Inc. (UOA) is a volunteer-based health organization dedicated to assisting people who have had or will have intestinal or urinary diversions. The UOA has over 400 chapters. They provide emotional support and rehabilitation programs, preoperative and postoperative visitation programs, and networks for parents of children with ostomies. They also produce several publications, such as the *Ostomy Quarterly* magazine.

WomenStories
1807 Elmwood Avenue
Buffalo, NY 14207
Telephone: 716-873-3689
Toll-free: 800-775-5790
Fax: 716-873-5361
Web site: www.womenstories.org

WomenStories, a nonprofit organization, benefits those who have been diagnosed with breast cancer and need the information and comfort that only other breast cancer survivors can provide. WomenStories produces a series of videos in which breast cancer survivors offer emotional support.

Young Survival Coalition
61 Broadway, Suite 2235
New York, NY 10006
Telephone: 646-257-3000
Toll-free: 877-972-1011
Fax: 646-257-3030
Web site: www.youngsurvival.org

The Young Survival Coalition is dedicated to the concerns and issues that are unique to women aged 40 and younger with breast cancer.

PROFESSIONAL MENTAL HEALTH ORGANIZATIONS

American Association for Marriage and Family Therapy
112 S. Alfred Street
Alexandria, VA 22314-3061
Telephone: 703-838-9808
Fax: 703-838-9805
Web site: www.aamft.org

The American Association for Marriage and Family Therapy (AAMFT) is the professional association for the field of marriage and family therapy. AAMFT provides referrals to local marriage and family therapists. They also provide educational materials to help couples live with illness and other issues related to families and health. AAMFT represents the professional interests of more than 50,000 marriage and family therapists throughout the United States, Canada, and abroad.

American Association of Pastoral Counselors
9504-A Lee Highway
Fairfax, VA 22031-2303
Telephone: 703-385-6967
Fax: 703-352-7723
E-mail: info@aapc.org
Web site: www.aapc.org

The American Association of Pastoral Counselors provides an online directory of Certified Pastoral Counselors across the nation. The organization's mission is to bring healing, hope, and wholeness to individuals, families, and communities by expanding and equipping spiritually grounded and psychologically informed care, counseling, and psychotherapy.

American Counseling Association
5999 Stevenson Avenue
Alexandria, VA 22304
Toll-free: 800-347-6647
Fax: 800-473-2329
Web site: www.counseling.org

The American Counseling Association (ACA) is a nonprofit professional and educational organization dedicated to the growth and enhancement of the counseling profession. The organization provides leadership training, publications, continuing education opportunities, and advocacy services to nearly 45,000 members. ACA helps counseling professionals develop their skills and expand their knowledge base. ACA provides information to consumers for how to locate a professional counselor through the National Board of Certified Counselors (www.nbcc.org/counselorfind) and other sources.

American Psychiatric Association
1000 Wilson Boulevard, Suite 1825
Arlington, VA 22209
Toll-free: 888-357-7924 (888-35-PSYCH)
Telephone: 703-907-7300
E-mail: apa@psych.org
Web site: www.psych.org

The American Psychiatric Association provides information on mental health and referrals. It represents more than 36,000 psychiatric physicians from the United States and around the world. Its member physicians work to ensure humane care and effective treatment for all persons with mental disorders, including intellectual developmental disorders and substance use disorders.

American Psychological Association
750 First Street, NE
Washington, DC 20002-4242
Toll-free: 800-374-2721
Telephone: 202-336-5500
Web site: www.apa.org

The American Psychological Association (APA) is a scientific and professional organization that represents psychology in the United States. Its mission is to advance the creation, communication, and application of psychological knowledge to benefit society and improve people's lives. The APA offers referrals to psychologists in local areas. They also provide information on family issues, parenting, and health. The APA has links to state psychological associations that may also provide local referrals: http://locator.apa.org

American Psychosocial Oncology Society
154 Hansen Road, Suite 201
Charlottesville, VA 22911
Toll-free: 866-276-7443
Telephone: 434-293-5350
Fax: 434-977-1856
Web site: www.apos-society.org

The American Psychosocial Oncology Society explores innovative methods to enhance the recognition and treatment of psychological, social, behavioral, and spiritual aspects of cancer. They provide clinical information, education, and a hotline for counseling and support services in order to promote the well-being of patients with cancer and families at all stages of disease. They also strive to raise the level of awareness of health professionals and the public about psychological, social, behavioral, and spiritual domains of care for patients with cancer.

American Society of Clinical Oncology
2318 Mill Road, Suite 800
Alexandria, VA 22314
Toll-free: 888-282-2552
Telephone: 571-483-1300
E-mail: membermail@asco.org
Web site: www.asco.org
CancerNet: www.peoplelivingwithcancer.org

The American Society of Clinical Oncology (ASCO) has information about cancer doctors, research, treatment, and patient care. The ASCO-sponsored *CancerNet* Web site provides information on types of cancer, coping, and patient support organizations.

Association of Oncology Social Work
100 North 20th Street, 4th Floor
Philadelphia, PA 19103
Telephone: 215-599-6093
Fax: 215-564-2175
E-mail: info@aosw.org
Web site: www.aosw.org

Oncology social work is the primary professional discipline that provides psychosocial services to cancer patients, their families, and caregivers. Oncology social workers connect patients and their families with community, state, national, and international resources. The Association of Oncology Social Work and its members work to increase awareness about the social, emotional, educational, and spiritual needs of cancer patients through research, writing, workshops and lectures, and collaborations with other patient advocacy groups and national and international oncology organizations whose primary focus is access to quality care for cancer patients.

National Association of Social Workers
750 First Street, NE, Suite 700
Washington, DC 20002-4241
Toll-free: 800-638-8799
Telephone: 202-408-8600
Web site: www.socialworkers.org

The National Association of Social Workers (NASW) is the largest membership organization of professional social workers in the world. The NASW Register of Clinical Social Workers, available on the Web site under "Find a Social Worker," is a resource members of the public can use to identify social workers who are qualified by education, experience, and credentials to provide mental health services.

Contributors Index